ENJOY IT!
Foods for healing and prevention

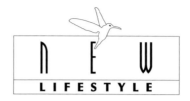

ENJOY IT!
Foods for healing and prevention

George D. Pamplona-Roger, M.D.
Doctor of Medicine, Specialist in General and Digestive Surgery

Author of the 'Encyclopedia of Medicinal Plants'
and the 'Encyclopedia of Foods and Their Healing Power'
published in English, French, German, Portuguese and Spanish

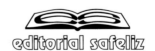

editorial safeliz

New Lifestyle
Enjoy it!

EDITORIAL TEAM

General Manager	**JONATHAN VALLS ESTEBANELL**	Edition	**RAQUEL CARMONA**
Administration	**ALEJO GOYA ROSET**		**MÓNICA DÍAZ**
Research & Development	**GEORGE D. PAMPLONA-ROGER**		**LUIS GONZÁLEZ SORIANO**
Editorial Coordination	**ELISABETH SANGÜESA ABENIA**		**JUAN F. SÁNCHEZ PEÑAS**
Production & Logistics	**MARTÍN GONZÁLEZ HUELMO**	Secretary	**Mª PILAR ARTAL**
		Layout, Design	**ISAAC CHÍA MAYOLAS**
		& Photography	**JOSÉ Mª WEINDL**
			JAVIER ZANUY

Printing   Ibergraphi 2002 – E-28830 San Fernando de Henares, Madrid, Spain

PRINTED IN THE EUROPEAN UNION

April 2005: Nineth print in English language of the Spanish edition

Copyright by © **editorial safeliz**
          Pradillo, 6 – Polígono Industrial La Mina
          E-28770 Colmenar Viejo, Madrid, Spain
          tel. [+34] 918 459 877 – fax [+34] 918 459 865
          e-mail: admin@safeliz.com – www.safeliz.com

Legal Deposit: M-16671-2005
          ISBN: 84-7208-130-3
          ISBN: 84-7208-100-1, Editorial Safeliz, original edition

CONTENTS

Now is the time

*E*VERYONE *agrees that health is something to be treasured. Developed countries have modern hospitals equipped with sophisticated medical equipment, emergency services ready to help when needed at any time, day or night, and numerous pharmaceutical products to treat almost any illness. All this has helped raise the health level of the population, as well as life expectancy and quality of life. Many illnesses which were fatal a few decades ago, can now be cured or alleviated.*

Nevertheless, certain health problems occur with increasing frequency despite technical progress in the world of medicine. Heart diseases, especially myocardial infarction, disturbances caused by the lack of circulation in the brain or the extremities, rheumatic and degenerative diseases, and above all, cancer, seem to be increasing every day. Isn't medical technology capable of detecting them early and dealing with them?

Actually, no. The most advanced medical technology and the best specialists cannot compensate for poor health habits. No matter how many coronary bypasses and heart trans-

Choose the best. Habit soon will make it pleasant for you.

PYTHAGORAS
Greek philosopher
and mathematician
6th century B.C.

plants are performed in a given country, its people will not be healthier or at less risk of heart attack. A healthful lifestyle with simple health habits can do much more for the health of its people than the most advanced medical technology.

This is recognized by those who are responsible for health in governments and public institutions. The National Institutes of Health in all western countries have launched a major program to slow the alarming increase in cancer. This is reflected in the ten points that make up the European Code Against Cancer. To lessen the incidence of this curse on society, we are urged to change our habits and adopt a more healthful lifestyle. Here are some examples:

✓ Don't smoke (Point No. 1)

✓ Control your consumption of alcohol (Point No. 2) (Preferably don't use any, according to the US National Academy of Sciences and the World Health Organization).

✓ Eat often fresh fruit and vegetables and cereals with high fiber content (Point No. 3)*

The illnesses with the highest mortality rate at present (heart disease and cancer) have much to do with lifestyle. And among all human activities eating undoubtedly has the greatest effect on health. At least 40% of all present diseases are related to diet. After breathing, eating is what we do most frequently during a lifetime.

With this book the publishers wish to place in your hands the result of the latest scientific research in the fields of preventive medicine and nutrition. The author has made his best effort to express in simple and easy-to-understand language that which can sometimes be difficult and complex.

This book on preventive medicine teaches how to live a healthful lifestyle and how to avoid illness before it comes. It is addressed primarily to healthy people rather than to the sick.

We thank Dr. Pere Llorca, who has a Master's degree in Nutrition and Health Education from Loma Linda University in California, for revising the text in harmony with the latest research in the field of health.

Today, as never before in history, we understand the secrets of healthful living. We have valuable information, scientifically documented, to improve our health. As never before, we know what foods we should eat to avoid the most serious illnesses of our times.

Never have there been better or more abundant reasons to adopt a **new** and better **lifestyle.** Enjoying this, as you will see in this book, is within the reach of everyone.

Now, is the best time to change to a new lifestyle. ENJOY IT!

THE EDITORS

---

* Point 5 in the first version of the Code.

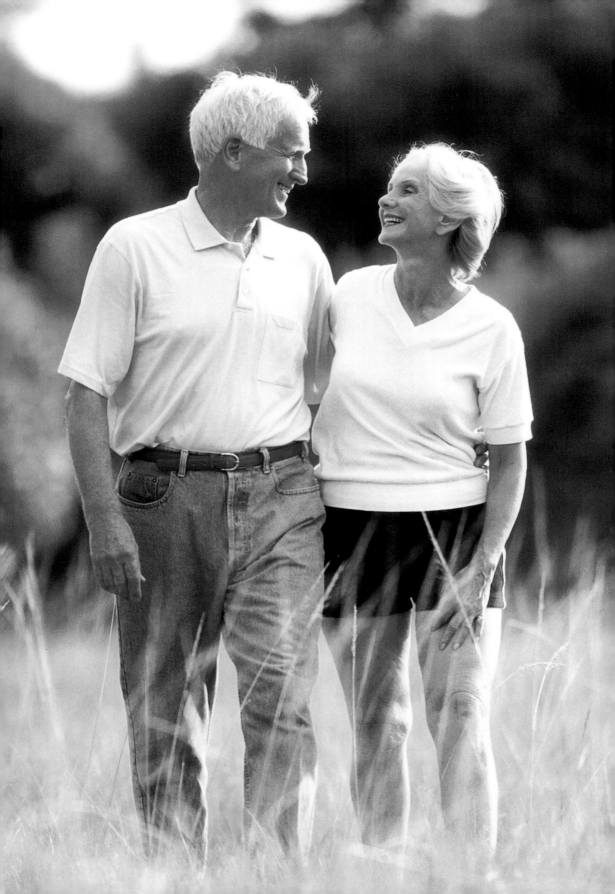

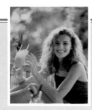

ENJOY IT!

Foods for healing and prevention

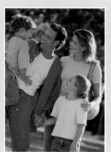

The basis for good health

Within the eight basic principles for the natural conservation of health, diet holds a significant position.

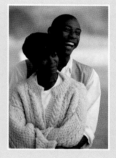

The elements that maintain health

The basic nutrients for health must not only be free from pollution and manipulation, but they must be of prime quality.

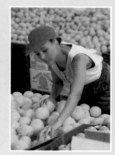

Vitamins, minerals, oligoelements, phytochemical elements, antioxidants

The latest discoveries that allow our quality of life to be improved and the ageing process to be delayed.

The adventure of rediscovering forgotten truths

The newest and the latest discoveries regarding health do not always mean progress and sometimes a step backwards could mean a giant step forward.

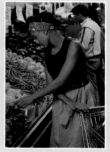

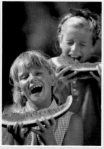

Simple and truly natural elements continue to be the best

The return to natural elements is worth it, but it has its secrets ... today placed within the reach of all readers.

OUTLINE
see "Contents", page 5

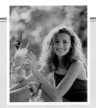

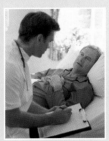

Suitable motivation is the best guarantee of success

Health, ecological, ethical reasons ...
To start practicing, with a good outlook for success,
a new lifestyle.

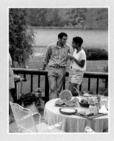

Never before have there been so many or such "good" reasons for the change

You can live without eating meat or fish ... and you live better,
food is savored more ... enjoying the most delicious dishes.

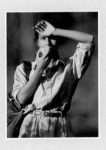

A new, healthy and balanced lifestyle

Balance is not formed by "eating a little of everything",
but by eating what is necessary and what is healthy
in suitable proportions.

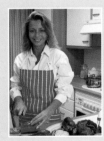

An important change made step by step ...

And each step in the right direction, with the certainty that is
inspired by knowing the goal beforehand, marching towards it in
accordance with safe, serious and scientifically proven indications.

Self-evaluation TESTS

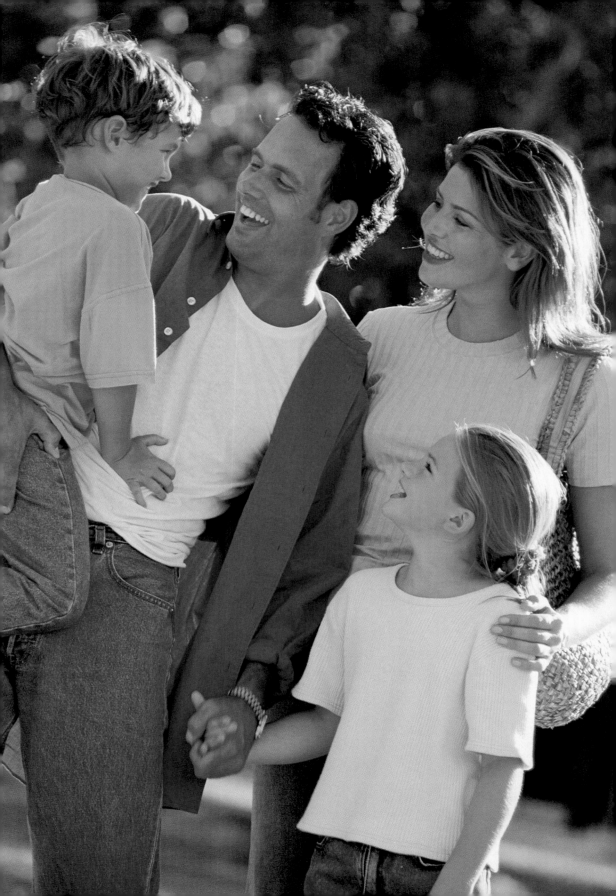

1

Eight Decisive Factors

"SOME PEOPLE seek to reach heaven," *Oliver Wendell Holmes* once said, "while making of earth a hell". He was referring to the habits involved in a healthy lifestyle, and not without irony. Generally throughout many years, the impression has been given that healthful habits are boring, difficult to implement, or just very unattractive. Many feel that to maintain a healthful lifestyle, a large number of "no's" must be put into effect.

Fortunately, however, this isn't so. Developing an interest in health and acquiring healthful habits may actually be both pleasant and creative. Applying a healthful lifestyle definitely does not make of earth a hell. Quite the opposite, there is actually an advantage in changing to a more healthful lifestyle.

Beyond eating, there are seven natural factors that are decisive in the maintenance of health. Their application is very simple. Making these factors the basis of your lifestyle can be very pleasant and gratifying.

> A healthy
> body is a guest.
> A sick body is
> a jailer.
>
> FRANCIS BACON
> English philosopher and politician
> 1561-1626

Eating

The beneficial effects of a **healthy diet,** as presented in this book, are *strengthened* when practiced with other health habits: **pure air, water, sunshine, physical exercise, rest, abstinence from toxic materials and a good mental attitude.** All these together form a great program for healthful living. To apply them enthusiastically will for you turn this earth into a little bit of heaven.

Eating is a *habit* which *affects* our *health more than anything else.* Not only the kind of food, but also the time and manner in which it is eaten, have a decided effect upon the organism. In this book the reader will find what is needed to eat adequately, pleasantly and healthfully.

Air

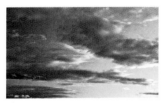

It is possible to live several weeks without food; several days without water; but we cannot live more than three or four minutes without breathing. The **oxygen** in the air is necessary for food to be burned in our cells to produce energy for living. And there is only one way to obtain this oxygen: by breathing.

We must **breathe well** and deeply. Furthermore it is necessary to breathe **pure air.** Good physical **posture** must be maintained, with the upper torso erect to facilitate breathing. Try to see to it that your **place of work** and your **bedroom** are always well ventilated. Remember that when someone smokes in an enclosed area, all who breathe this contaminated air are also "smoking."

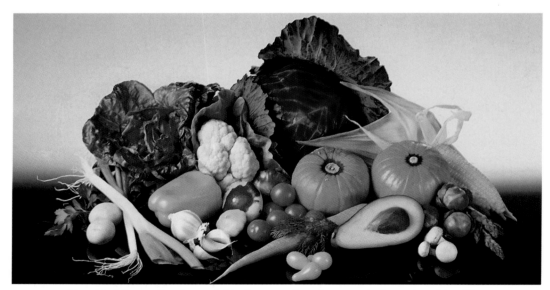

Good habits are fundamental in the practice of a more balanced and healthy new lifestyle. Fortunately, nature provides a great symphony of colors, scents and flavors making the change pleasant.

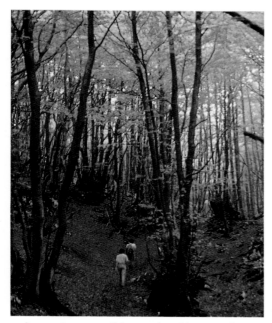

As much as possible we should go out into the country and take advantage of the opportunity to breath pure air. The total organism is stimulated by deep breathing.

ter so that the feces are not too dry or hard, causing strain; the **skin** needs water to maintain itself firm and healthy; and even the **bones** should contain an adequate proportion of water to maintain their elasticity and hardness.

We need to apply **water externally** (for personal hygiene) as well as **internally.** **Every day** try to drink at least **six glasses** of water between meals (more in the summer). Drink two glasses **before breakfast,** making sure they are not too cold. This will cleanse the stomach from all the mucus that accumulates during the night. Drink one or two more glasses of water before the noon meal, and another one or two glasses before the evening meal. **Choose water above all other drinks.**

Water applied externally has a great healing power, known from ancient times. The techniques of **hydrotherapy,** whether applied in a public place or at home, such as jets, wrappings, sauna and different kinds of baths, may lessen or even heal many illnesses. Resort to using water as much as possible, even though it may be only once in a while to take a hot bath with bath salts, and relax before going to sleep at night.

It is always well to start the day by taking some deep breaths in an open area. Take advantage of every opportunity to go outdoors and breathe deeply. **Respiration** is the *first function* of life. Your brain and your entire organism will function better if you breathe the purest air possible.

The abundant use of water, both internally and externally, is a good health habit which may prevent many diseases and even contribute to their healing.

Water

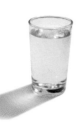

Water is the universal solvent of living matter. Around **60%** of our **body** is made up of water. **Kidneys** need water to filter the blood and eliminate unneeded substances through the urine; the **digestive system** needs wa-

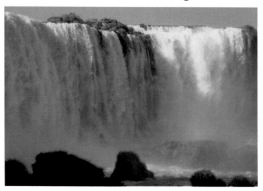

The Sun

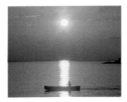

The sun is the main source of energy for our planet. Solar light is **absolutely necessary** for **life** and for the maintenance of **health.** Its presence produces **vitamin D** in the skin. Ultraviolet radiation in sunlight serves as a **disinfectant** capable of destroying numerous pathogenic germs. Furthermore, it stimulates all the vital processes and serves as a tonic to the organism. **Where sunshine enters there is life and health.** It has been proven that in winter, when whole days go by without sunshine, the frequency of nervous depression increases.

Nevertheless the use of the sun must be **controlled,** since the **layer of ozone** that covers the earth and filters the solar rays (especially ultraviolet) is decreasing. This has led to more intense solar radiation, which is affecting the surface of the earth. It has never been good, and especially bad today, to spend many hours exposing the body to the sun.

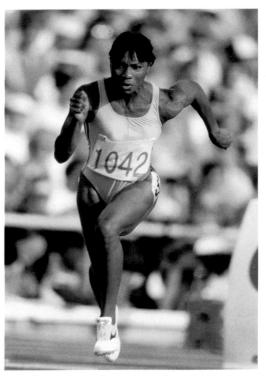

Physical exercise, adapted to the possibilities and age of each individual, is never a waste of time but an unavoidable necessity in order to maintain ourselves fit and healthy.

Physical Exercise

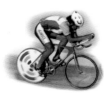

Our body is designed for movement. Contrary to what happens when something is built by man, **inactivity** in the body leads to *more deterioration* than does **exercise.** It has been demonstrated that persons who dedicate at least four periods of forty minutes each to physical exercise every week run a *smaller risk* of having a **heart attack** or **circulatory diseases.** Exercise combats **arterial hypertension,** *prevents* **obesity** and *keeps* the entire organism in **good condition.**

The best physical exercise for everyone—which may be done without restriction—is walking. *"All of us have two doctors: the right leg and the left leg,"* says an ancient proverb.

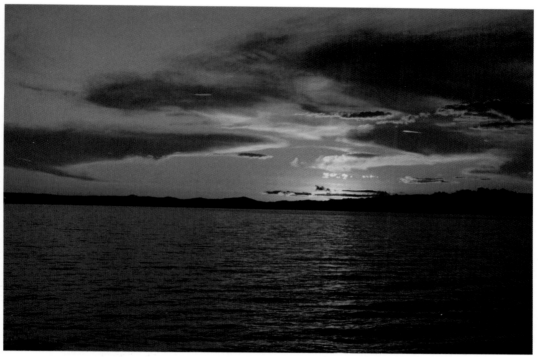

All nature follows cycles of activity and rest, in which our bodies also participate. Respect for them is a decisive factor in our mental and physical well-being.

Rest

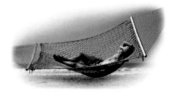

It is also a known fact that most of heart attacks take place between 9 and 12 p.m. And this almost always occurs after an stressful day, during which tobacco and coffee have been generously used; until the body's limit of resistance has been reached, and the attack occurs.

We must make sure that our rest is a **restoring** one. As we sleep, the neurons cleanse themselves of metabolic waste which has accumulated during the day. All of our body cells need a sufficient period of rest each day. This should be regular—a *minimum* of **seven hours** for adults.

But aside from daily rest, our bodies need other periods of rest: the **weekly** (at least one day per week) and the **annual.** There have been occasions when an effort has been made to change the length of the week. During the French Revolution, moved by a rationalist philosophy, they tried to set up a week of ten days. Wouldn't this be logical? But the effort failed. There is something within the human being which makes a period of rest necessary every seven days. It is a biological need, undoubtedly set up by the Creator. Regular rest is a good health habit.

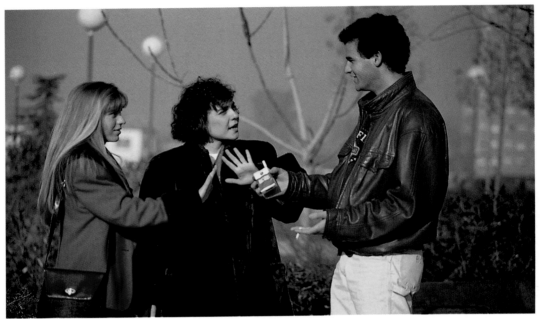

Abstinence of all that may be harmful, and moderate use of that which is good, are also decisive factors for our well-being. Health is not the result of chance, but depends on our life-style.

Abstinence From Toxics

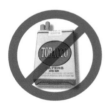

The human being is the only being which voluntarily destroys its health with toxic substances. The harmfulness of coffee, alcoholic beverages, and above all tobacco and dangerous drugs, has been sufficiently demonstrated. If we wish to have a vigorous and healthful mind, we must avoid any substance which may alter the delicate mechanisms of our brain. **Addictive stimulants** (caffeine, nicotine, alcohol, cocaine, etc.) cause our organism to operate under forced conditions, which leads to early deterioration and disease.

The use of tobacco and alcoholic beverages is the main avoidable cause of disease throughout the world, according to the World Health Organization. This organization defines **health** as *total **physical, mental** and **social** well-being, which takes in much more than simply the absence of sickness.*

Health is incompatible with the use of drugs, whether legal or illegal, which makes no difference to our cells. Their use is initiated under the pretense of feeling better, but at the end they must be taken in order not to feel worse. To avoid the use of these toxic substances is one of the best decisions which may be made to promote a happy and healthful life.

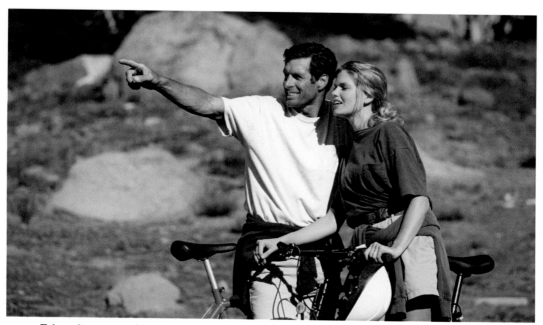

Take advantage of every opportunity to relax as you contemplate nature. At times raise your eyes heavenward. Believe and trust that there is a superior Power who is above all. To believe in something and to have hope in something promotes a good mental attitude and positively affects the whole body.

Good Mental attitude

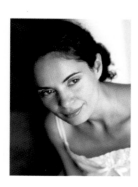

Acquire the habit of taking all things calmly; of not worrying about yourself; of not holding grudges against others or yourself; of confidently smiling as you face the problems of life.

It has often been demonstrated that an attitude of mental equilibrium is an *essential* factor to **health.** Did you know that some studies show that cancer more frequently affects those who are depressed or ill-humored?

To gain this mental peace in the midst of the many tensions and problems presented to us by modern life is not an easy task. Many seek this in faith, finding that the reading of the Gospels, as well as prayer and private meditation, are like a glass of fresh water to their agitated nervous systems.

Confidence and **faith** may do much toward obtaining a good mental attitude, and a **spirit of peace,** which will benefit both mental and physical **health.** This comes because the believer lives in the firm hope of a better future, and with the conviction that there is Someone over him who understands and loves him.

A good mental disposition and peace of the spirit decisively influence the good functioning of our bodies.

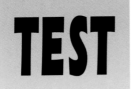

TEST

Evaluate Your Lifestyle

Daily habits of life such as eating, working or the use of free time exert a powerful influence upon our health. More than heredity or luck, our health depends on lifestyle.

The questions below are included to help you evaluate to what degree your habits and way of life are favoring your health and your expectations of life, or may be harming them.

Positive Habits

Points

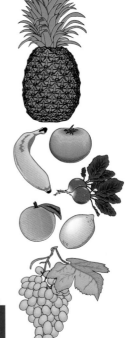

I eat at least three pieces of fruit each day 2

Each day I eat at least one plate of raw
    vegetables (salad) 2

I regularly eat whole cereals 2

I use olive, seed or vegetable oils 2

I maintain a regular schedule of meals 2

Every day I breathe deeply several times 2

I drink 4 to 8 glasses of water every day 2

I have a normal bowel movement daily 2

I spend at least one half hour per day in the
    open air 2

I try to go into the country at least once a week 2

I engage in some physical exercise each week 2

I regularly sleep seven hours per night 2

I rest and relax at least one day per week 2

I maintain a good mental attitude 2

Total positive points ....

Negative Habits

Points

I snack between meals	1
I eat meat more than four times per week	1
I eat candy, pastries and sweets every day	1
I habitually eat sausages, pork, lard, or cream	1
I eat smoked products	1
I am overweight	1
I live in a polluted city	1
I frequently spend sleepless nights	1
My work hours are quite irregular	1
I smoke	1
I smoke over one pack of cigarettes each day	1
I drink alcoholic beverages every week	1
I drink liquors (cognac, whiskey, etc.)	1
I drink more than two cups of coffee each day	1

Total negative points ....

Positive minus negative points =

Results

From -14 to -1 points: You urgently need to change your lifestyle. Your short range expectancy is not good, and it won't be long until you will suffer a serious illness, if you are not already undergoing one.

From 0 to 13 points: You should seriously review some of your life habits which are cutting down on your health and vitality. You may obtain great results with a few changes. Try it!

From 14 to 20 points: You are doing everything quite well, and are surely enjoying good health, but there are still several points where you may improve. Continue as you are doing and try to enrich your lifestyle with new healthful habits.

From 21 to 28 points: You are carrying on a healthful lifestyle, and are enjoying the results. Help others who wish to improve their health habits, but be careful! Do this tactfully and considerately.

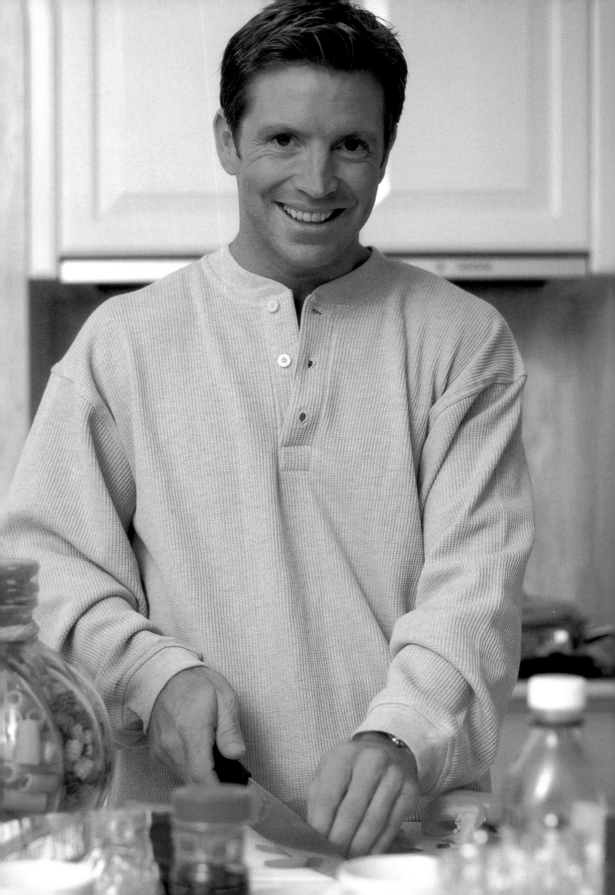

The Value of Nutrition

2

EATING is undoubtedly the habit which exerts the **greatest influence** upon the **health** of individuals. And there is a reason, for the habit of eating repeats itself constantly throughout life. **Dr. Osler,** famous Canadian physician, said that 90% of all sicknesses, leaving aside infections and accidents, are related to diet.

Eating is a *voluntary and conscious process,* and therefore it can be **educated.** It depends upon the free choice of the individual. Therefore a change to more healthful eating habits demands that an individual be thoroughly convinced.

On the other hand, **nutrition** is *involuntary and unconscious.* It covers all the processes and transformation that foods undergo in the body, until they have been thoroughly assimilated. Under normal conditions, if there are no pathological problems, good nourishment should be equivalent to a good nutritional state.

> Eat little,
> my friend Sancho,
> and even less
> at supper,
> for the stomach is the
> place where
> good health and life
> are forged.
>
> **DON QUIXOTE**
> Miguel de Cervantes
> 1547-1616

In recent years, nutritionists have emphasized four fundamental aspects of foods:

1. Food Hygiene

Hygiene, or the *absence of pathogenic germs* which may provoke infectious diseases in the consumer, is a priority among the nutritional experts and health authorities. **Salmonellosis,** a very serious form of gastroenteritis, causes serious health problems produced by *Salmonella*. **Botulism** is poisoning caused by the use of poorly canned goods, produced by the microorganism *Clostridium botulinum;* and the summer **gastroenteritis** through foods contaminated with staphylococcus, among other diseases.

Nevertheless, although toxic infections are still resulting from contaminated food, we know how these infections are caused, and how we may avoid them.

In the light of present knowledge concerning nourishment and nutrition, we cannot be satisfied in knowing that a certain food has no pathogenic germs or toxins, to consider it appropriate to use as food. Food hygiene is indispensable, but not enough to determine its quality. Today we know that if a piece of meat or an egg are completely free of microorganisms, this is no reason to consider them adequate, for example, for someone who must control his cholesterol.

2. Calories

In the nutrition manuals of the recent past, special emphasis was given to the number of calories that must be consumed daily. A diet is adequate, it was said, if it included sufficient calories to cover the needs of the body. It's to understand that this may have been true in the times when there was a scarcity of foods, as is unfortunately still happening in the third world. At present, however, in the western world, the problem is an excess of calories, rather than too few.

The quality and value of a diet cannot be measured only by all the calories that it furnishes, but rather by the nourishment that it provides. It is not a problem of quantity, but quality. For example:

- **Refined carbohydrates** (flour or white rice, for example) contain practically the same number of calories as whole foods, but their quality is much less.

- **White sugar** has practically the same number of calories as brown sugar or honey, but is greatly lacking in vitamins and minerals, which means that it is not adequate for habitual or large-scale use.

- **Lean meat** and **soybeans** furnish a much similar quantity of calories, nevertheless their adequacy for a healthful diet is very different.

3. Proteins

There are still some specialists (diminishing in number) who believe that a diet, to be correct from a nutritional point of view, should contain a high amount of protein, and that this should be largely of animal origin. Nevertheless the recommended amount of protein in the diet has been diminishing for several decades. Twenty or thirty years ago it was recommended that an adult should include at least one gram of protein daily for each kilo of body weight. And there were some who proposed 1.2 to 1.5 grams per kilo per day. At present, a report of a study group of the WHO on nutrition, says that ***0.75 grams*** of protein ***per kilo*** of weight each ***day*** is sufficient for an adult (56 grams per day for a man or woman weighing 70 kilos [154 lb]).[1] Today we know that an excess of protein in the diet is related to rheumatic diseases, osteoporosis, kidney damage, excess of uric acid, and a shorter life span.

Previously it was thought that proteins of animal origin were indispensable, and that diet lacked sufficient nutrition if it did not contain abundant animal proteins. But it has been proven that, thanks to the phenome-

The Masai are Tanzanian and Kenyan herders whose food base is meat and milk. They drink the blood of their animals. This diet which is rich in protein results in great and rapid growth. But they also become ill and die sooner than other peoples who eat a diet based on vegetables.

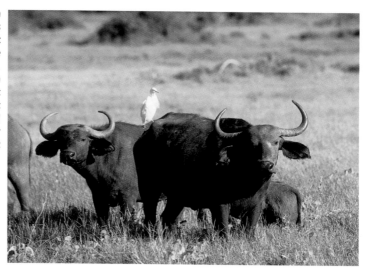

non of **supplementation,** a sufficient quantity of proteins can be obtained by **combining vegetable proteins,** as if they were of animal origin.

So the quality of diet does not depend, as thought in previous times, on the quantity of proteins, or their origin, but rather on the use of a sufficient **variety** of **healthful foods** (see page 61).

4. The Effect Upon Growth

This is another of the parameters which have been used up to several years ago to measure the value of a diet. The more the growth, they thought, the better the diet. And they placed as examples peoples who attained great stature such as the Masai of Tanzania and Kenya, who have as their basis a diet of meat, milk and blood (they have the custom of drinking the blood of their animals), while other neighboring peoples like

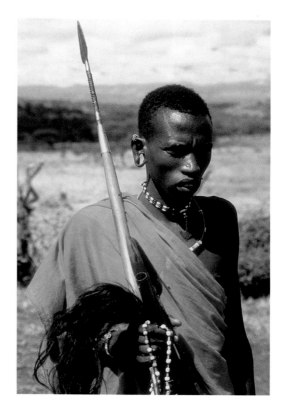

1. WHO, Technical Report Series, No. 797, (*Diet, Nutrition, and the Prevention of Chronic Diseases*). Report of a WHO Study Group. Geneva, World Health Organization, 1990, page 168.

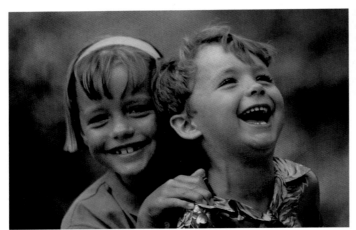

It has been demonstrated that total vegetarian children grow slower than those who eat meat, although they eventually grow as tall or taller than the latter.

the Kikuyos, who have only access to vegetable proteins, are shorter and very thin. What was not known is that those who grow more quickly also become ill and die sooner. Hyperproteinic and hypercaloric foods that are given to children in developed countries, which result in faster growth, may have serious repercussions in adolescents and adults: obesity and greater risk of diabetes and arteriosclerosis, among others.

Therefore, the mere fact that a diet results in greater and faster growth, does not imply that it is good. Of course, insufficient growth may be due to a deficient diet; but notable growth, is not always synonymous with a balanced diet.

Types of Diets

Based on Meats. Meat and **fish** are its basic components. This type of diet results in an **excess** of **proteins** and **fats** and a lack of carbohydrates and fiber, with negative repercussions upon health, for example: an excess of uric acid and cholesterol, intestinal putrefaction, and a greater possibility of cardiac problems (heart attacks, angina pectoris, and cancer).

Omnivorous. It is the diet followed by the greater number of people, who eat a great assortment of foods including an ample amount of **animal** and **vegetable** products.

Ovolactovegetarian. An ovolactovegetarian diet excludes meat, fish and fowl. It includes eggs and milk products in small or moderate quantities, and above all, vegetables: cereals, fruit, garden products (vegetables, legumes and tubers). It is recognized that this provides a **satisfactory diet** from the nutritional point of view, and that it is **easy to follow,** is appropriate for **children,** and has **great advantages** over the omnivorous diet.

Adults should limit their use of eggs to three per week, and milk products should be non-fat in order to avoid a large intake of cholesterol.

Lactovegetarian. It includes only milk and dairy products as sources of food origi-

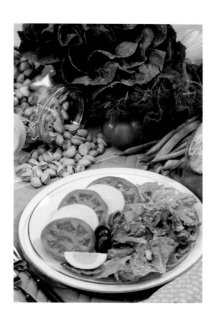

nating from animals. It is equally **satisfactory** in nutritional value. The proteins in the milk complement and enrich vegetable proteins, so that it is not difficult to obtain the essential amino acids. It is preferable that especially adults should use low or non-fat milk products.

Strict vegetarian (vegan). It includes only vegetable foods, omitting all animal products. It provides all the necessary nutrients, including proteins, providing that precautions are taken at the time that **selection** and **combination** of foods are made (see pages 61 and 140). The strict vegetarian may need vitamin B_{12} supplements.

This kind of diet presents interesting **advantages** when compared to the omnivorous diet (page 115), and provides the **best results** in the **prevention** and **treatment** of **chronic degenerative diseases** such as arteriosclerosis (circulatory problems, angina pectoris, myocardial attacks), rheumatic diseases and cancer, among others.

In speaking of a strict vegetarian diet, we are not referring to some unbalanced and deficient diets, such as the zen-macrobiotic (which lead only to eating cereals) or the raw diets (in which only raw foods are eaten), but we refer to an exclusively vegetarian diet, varied and satisfactory from the nutritional viewpoint.

Diet and Beauty

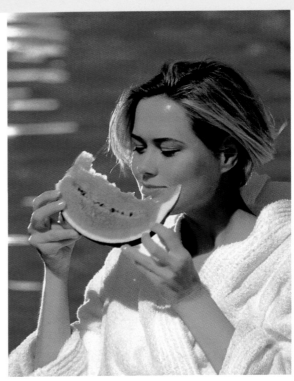

A balanced diet which includes fruit, cereals and vegetables, provides vitamins and minerals which are indispensable for the good condition of the skin, and for a real beauty treatment "from the inside out."

Diet greatly affects our general appearance. An adequate diet may even make us appear more attractive, as it increases the firmness and glow of the skin, face and body in general. These are some of the signs of adequate nutrition which have much to do with the pleasing appearance of our bodies.

The Skin

Many women try to solve the problem of oily or scaly skin by using products which are applied externally, without taking into consideration the fact that skin cells are formed, as are others, from foods that are ingested.

Eating an **abundant quantity** of **fruit and vegetables** which provide vitamins A and C, the elimination of foods overloaded with spices, abstinence from alcoholic beverages, and replacing the use of animal fats with vegetable oils, may be sufficient to restore health to an abused skin. Let us not forget that a **balanced diet** is the **best beauty treatment.**

Hair and Nails

Hair and nails are body tissues; for this reason a deficient diet may lead to broken fingernails, with small white spots, and to dry, colorless and dull hair. Certain diseases that affect the hair such as seborrhea and dandruff at times may be aggravated by an inadequate diet.

To have silky and shiny **hair,** and resistant and well-formed nails, we should have a diet rich in **vitamins** and **minerals** (particularly **trace elements**) which may be found mainly in fruits and vegetables. **Iron** and **silicon** are two minerals whose lack will especially affect the firmness of the **nails.**

The Eyes

The nutritional condition of a person can sometimes be seen in the appearance of the eyes. Clear, shiny eyes, with no redness, and no scales on the eyelids, are an indication of good nutrition. There are deficiencies in **vitamins A** and **B₂** that are perceived in the eyes: a loss of vision where there is little light, falling and dryness of the eyebrows, redness, etc. The so-called colored vegetables (peppers, carrots, tomatoes) are a good source of Vitamin A in the form of **carotene** (provitamin).

Smiles

A smile is a sign of good nutrition, and magnifies body beauty. Nevertheless a smile may not be attractive if it does not reveal **healthy teeth.** To help teeth grow

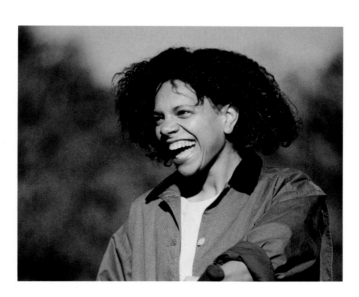

strong and well formed, it is necessary to combine three factors: periodic **vigilance, hygiene,** and adequate **diet.** Foods rich in **calcium,** such as dry fruit or milk provide the needed ingredients to form healthy teeth. On the other hand, food and drinks that are laden with **sugar** are the **worst enemies** of teeth, for they favor the development of caries. Snacking or eating between meals often is the prescription for getting **cavities** in your teeth.

Weight

Adequate weight is needed to maintain an attractive body, and is an indication of correct diet and good health. In order to maintain weight within correct limits, it is well to base the **diet** on **vegetarian** foods: fruit, cereals (grains) and garden products. It is very difficult to find a **fat** vegetarian. As is mentioned on page 164, the abundant use of fats, especially those of animal origin, is one of the most important factors in obesity caused by food.

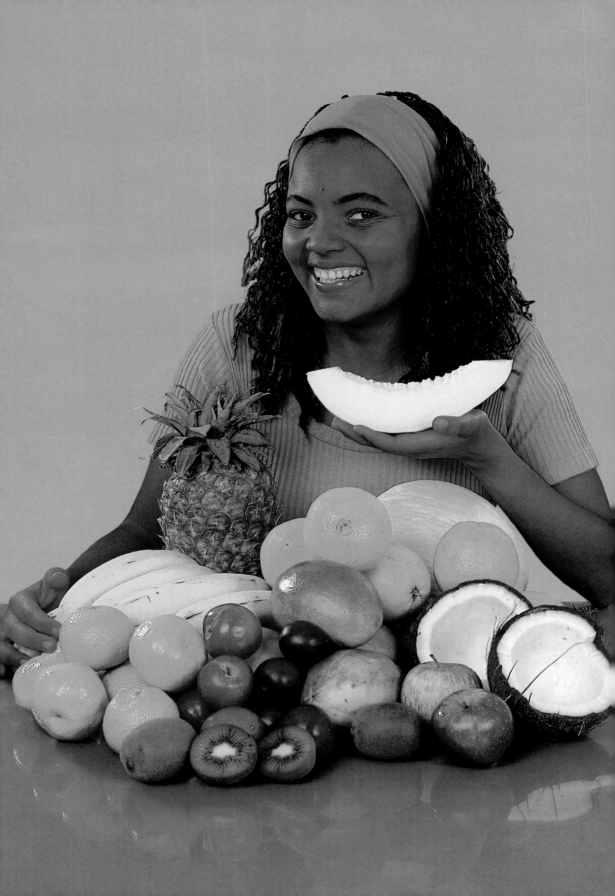

3

Why Do We Eat?

FROM THE MOMENT that food is chewed and swallowed, until it is utilized as energy or for the building up of the body, it undergoes several phases: **digestion, absorption,** and **metabolism.**

1. Digestion

Foods must be transformed so that the body may take advantage of the nutritive substances which they have. And digestion is exactly this process of transformation which is initiated in the mouth, and which causes changes, both physical and chemical, in the food structure.

The object of digestion is to break down the principal nutrients (carbohydrates, fats and proteins) into more simple chemical substances which may be passed to the blood, and thus be used by all the cells in the organism:

> May your food be your medicine and your medicine be your food.
>
> **HIPPOCRATES,**
> Greek physician,
> 5th century B.C.

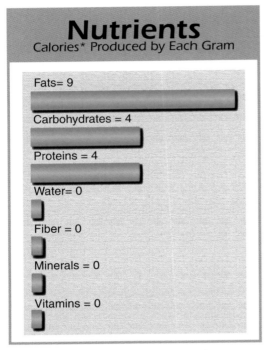

Nutrients
Calories* Produced by Each Gram

Fats= 9

Carbohydrates = 4

Proteins = 4

Water= 0

Fiber = 0

Minerals = 0

Vitamins = 0

*They are, in fact, kilocalories (see page 185).

- All the assimilable complex **carbohydrates** are transformed into *glucose.*
- All the **fats** are transformed into *glycerol* and *fatty acids.*
- All the **proteins** are transformed into *amino acids.*

Finally a mixture of glucose, glycerol and fatty acids remain in the intestines, as well as the **vitamins** and **minerals** which need no transformation.

2. Absorption

Through the lining of the small intestine, especially in its latter sections (jejunum and ileum), the following elemental **nutrients** are passed to the blood: glucose, glycerol, fatty acids, and amino acids, as well as **vitamins, minerals** and **water.** This is an active process, by which the organism regulates the absorption of nutritive substances according to the needs.

3. Metabolism

Once the nutrients enter the blood, they reach all the cells of the organism, where they are used (metabolized) to perform various functions:

Body Growth

Let us imagine a child who weights 3 kilos (6.6 lb) at birth who develops normally until he reaches the weight of 60 kilos (132 lb) at the age of 18. Well, those 57 kilos (125 lb) that the body has gained come from foods. The **minerals** which make up the skeleton (especially **calcium** and **phosphorus),** and the **amino acids** coming from proteins, are the nutrients which collaborate most in the development of the body, since they make up the basic structure of the organism.

Bananas are one of the fresh fruits that provide a good source of energy, because of their high content of carbohydrates (22%).

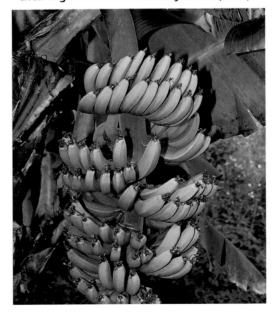

Nutrients Which Can Not Be Substituted

They are those which the organism is incapable of synthesizing from other chemical components, and this requires that they come from the outside.

Essential Amino Acids

They are a part of **proteins,** whether they be of animal or vegetable origin (see page 58). There are certain amino acids which the organism may obtain from the **essential amino acids,** but the latter **cannot be substituted.**

Essential Fatty Acids

These are the **polyunsaturated** fatty acids (linoleic and linolenic) which are found above all in **vegetable oils** and oily **dried foods,** especially in nuts (see page 52).

Vitamins and Minerals

These are found in all foods, especially in vegetables (see pages 65, 81).

Water

It is found in all foods but in a quantity insufficient to provide daily needs. Because of this, **6 to 8 cups** of water should be taken **daily,** a quantity which in summer time may need to be doubled, or even more (see page 15).

Fiber

Fiber is found **only** in **plant foods,** especially in whole grains, fruit and garden products (see page 43).

Though it is not a nutrient in the strictest sense, because it cannot be assimilated, it is **indispensable** for the good functioning of the organism.

Aside from the growth which only lasts to the age of 18 or 20, there is a permanent **repair** process and **substitution** of certain organic tissues: the skin, the hair, and the nails, for example, are renewed permanently. The mucosa material which lines the interiors of the hollow organs, are also subject to a permanent process of **renewal.** For example, the linings of the stomach change every 3 or 4 days, and that which covers the interior of the uterus changes on an average of every 28 days. Erythrocytes of the blood (red corpuscles) renew themselves every three months.

The materials for the permanent reconstruction of our organism also come from the food that we eat each day, especially **minerals** and the **proteins.**

Production of Energy

All of the vital processes require energy. Life itself is a permanent and uninterrupted user of energy. Foods are actually the **fuel** that provides energy needed for life.

One of the basic laws that governs the function of matter, known as the first principle of thermodynamics, states that "*energy is neither created nor destroyed, but only*

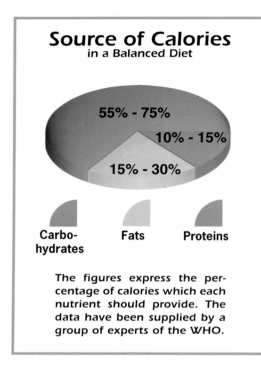

Source of Calories
in a Balanced Diet

55% - 75%

10% - 15%

15% - 30%

Carbo-   Fats   Proteins
hydrates

The figures express the percentage of calories which each nutrient should provide. The data have been supplied by a group of experts of the WHO.

transforms itself." So the food supplies chemical energy (which ultimately is derived from the sun) which our organism transforms into **electric** energy (for the functioning of the nervous system), to **caloric** energy (to maintain the body temperature) or to **mechanical** energy (to allow movement).

The nutrients that the body uses as fuel, in order to produce energy when they are burned with oxygen, come from carbohydrates, fats, and proteins.

- **Carbohydrates** (**starch** from cereals and tubers, and **sugars** from fruits) are the ***main* fuels** of the body, and this is practically their only function. All are finally transformed into **glucose,** a process which takes place above all in the liver. When glucose is burned (metabo-

lized), it produces approximately four calories per gram.

- **Fatty acids** come from the digestion of fats, and are used by the body as a rich source of energy (approximately nine calories for each gram burned). The excess fats left over because the body does not need them for energy are deposited in the tissues in the form of **body fat.**

- **Proteins** are designed primarily for ***growth*** and ***repair*** of the organic tissues. But the excess **amino acids** are burned to take advantage of their **energy** (approximately four calories per gram).

Specific Functions

A motor may be well structured, and the tank may be full of fuel, but without the spark from the spark plugs, it will not function. In the same way the body, aside from an adequate structure (minerals and proteins) and fuel (carbohydrates, fats, and also proteins), needs a spark which will unleash chemical reactions necessary for combustion. This spark is provided by **vitamins** and some minerals (**trace elements,** also called **oligoelements**) that act as ***catalysts,*** that is to say, as agents which unleash or facilitate the many chemical transformations which take place in our cells.

Vitamins and trace elements are neither building nor combustion materials, but are indispensable, in small quantities, for the operation of the body.

Transformation of Some Main Nutrients into Others

Nutrients may be transformed into others, according to the body needs and the peculiarities of the metabolism of each individual. **Carbohydrates** that are broken down into ***glucose*** may be transformed into ***fat*** (it is well known that starch fattens). Also **fatty acids** or **carbohydrates** (glucose) can be transformed into ***amino acids*** (but ***not*** the ***essential*** ones).

Laws for a Good Diet

The Law of Quantity

The amount of food introduced daily into the body should be **sufficient** to cover the needs of the organism, providing **energy**, and substances needed for **growth** and **maintenance** of our tissues and organs.

A diet is adequate when it allows the individual to fully perform the functions of:

✓ **growth**

✓ **reproduction**

✓ **occupation**

✓ **mental** activity and

✓ maintenance of **weight** in the adult.

The Law of Quality

Diet should be complete and varied in its make-up, so that these necessary substances will be provided to the body:

✓ **carbohydrates**

✓ **fats** (lipids)

✓ **proteins**

✓ **vitamins**

✓ **minerals**

✓ **water** and

✓ vegetable **fiber**

The Law of Balance

A **correct ratio** must be maintained between the various substances that provide energy as a part of the food supply (carbohydrates, fats and proteins).

- **Carbohydrates:** Should provide between **55%** and **75%** of the total calories, which would indicate that for a diet of 2,000 calories, between 1,100 and 1,500 calories should be in the form of carbohydrates. This implies a daily ingestion of 275 to 375 grams of carbohydrates.

- **Fats:** Should not exceed **30%** of the total calories ingested daily, and the largest part should be of **plant origin.** This presupposes a maximum of 66 grams of fats daily for an average diet of 2,000 calories.

- **Proteins:** Should make up **10%** to **15%** of the needed calories. This means that for a diet of 2,000 calories, there should be between 200 to 300 calories in the form of protein, which can be obtained with 50 to 75 grams of protein each day.

The Law of Adequacy

The choice, preparation and quantity of foods should be adequate to the **weight, age,** and **physical condition** of the individual as well as to the kind of work or **activity** that he performs.

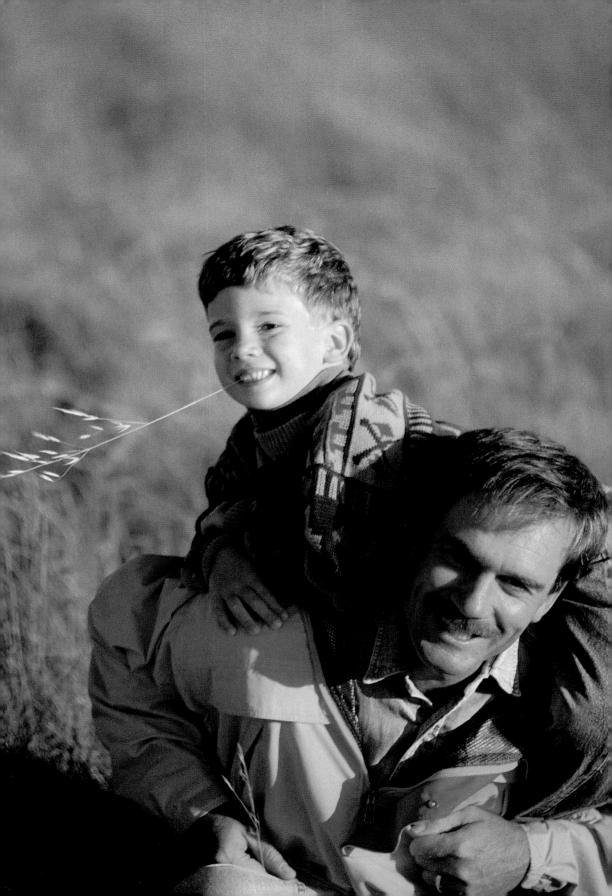

4

Carbohydrates

CARBOHYDRATES are also called **glucinums** because of their pronounced sweetness (the word *glucinum* comes from the Greek root *gluco*, sweet). They are the *main* source of **energy** for all the functions of the body, and provide **calories** *rapidly*.

Their molecules contain only **carbon**, **hydrogen**, and **oxygen** atoms. According to the size of the molecule, carbohydrates are classified into three groups: **monosaccharides**, **disaccharides**, and **polysaccharides**. The first two are also called **sugars**.

Chemical Composition

Monosaccharides

Are composed of only one molecule, and may be assimilated and absorbed directly and rapidly by the body. The most common monosaccharides found in nature are **glucose** or dextrose and **fructose** or levulose. Both are composed of the same atoms and

> If you want to be as strong as an ox, eat what the ox eats, but don't eat the ox.
>
> **EDWARD NELSON**
> Contemporary physician

only differ by their distribution within the molecule. Glucose and fructose are found in all fruits and in honey.

Disaccharides

Are **carbohydrates** formed by *two* **monosaccharide *molecules*.** To be able to be used by the body, the disaccharides have to be divided into their basic molecules, a task which is carried on by **enzymes** during the process of digestion. The most common disaccharides are:

- **Saccharose** (sucrose) or sugar cane, which is also found in beets, bananas, pineapple and in many other fruits. It is made up of a combination of a glucose molecule and a fructose molecule, which

upon binding loses one molecule of water.

glucose + fructose = sucrose + water

- **Maltose** which is found mainly in malt found in barley, as well as in other cereals. It is made up of two molecules of glucose.
- **Lactose,** which is found in the milk of mammals in the proportion of 40 grams per liter in cow milk, and between 50 and 60 in human milk. Its molecule is the result of the combination of two monosaccharides: glucose and galactose.

Polysaccharides

Are *complex* **carbohydrates** whose molecule is formed by the union of many

CARBOHYDRATES
daily needs (WHO)

	Percent of total energy required	In an average diet of 2,000 calories this is equivalent to	
Total carbohydrates			
Lower limit	55 %	1,100 calories	275 grams
Upper limit	75 %	1,500 calories	375 grams
Respect specific types of carbohydrates			
Complex carbohydrates (starch)			
Lower limit	50 %	1,000 calories	250 grams
Upper limit	70 %	1,400 calories	350 grams
Simple refined carbohydrates (white sugar)			
Lower limit	0 %	0 calories	0 grams
Upper limit	10 %	200 calories	50 grams
Fiber			
Lower limit	–	–	16 grams
Upper limit	–	–	24 grams

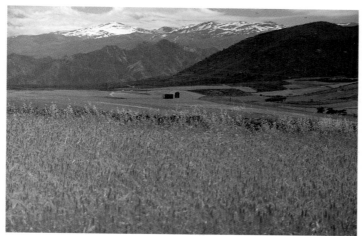

Wheat is undoubtedly the most important cereal for human consumption. Its great capacity for adaptation makes it possible to be cultivated in Siberia as well as in tropical regions. The whole wheat grain contains around 60% of complex carbohydrates (starch), around 13% of proteins and 2% of fats, in addition to vegetable fiber and various vitamins and minerals.

monosaccharides, generally glucose. They are mostly found in cereal grains (wheat, rice, barley, corn, etc.) as well as in roots and tubers (potatoes, turnips, etc.) There are three types of **polysaccharides** of complex carbohydrates:

- **Starch:** Its molecule is formed by long chains of glucose molecules, united in a special way. It is found in seeds, roots, tubers, leaves and fruit, and is the principal component of **flour.** Starch is produced *only* in the **vegetable** kingdom. Animals take advantage of starch by breaking down, during the process of digestion, the glucose molecules that compose it. This process is carried on by enzymes called **amylase,** which are secreted with the saliva, and above all in the pancreas. Starch is the most important food energy reserve in the vegetable kingdom.

- **Dextrines**: Are fragments of the starch molecule which result from the action of the amylase. These enzymes first break down starch into small fragments before completely separating all the glucose molecules which compose it. So it can be said that dextrines are *predigested* *starches.* In dextrinized bread or cereals, for example, the starch in flour is subjected to the chemical action of the amylase, enzymes which partially break down the

large chain of glucose molecules. This results in *easier* **digestion,** for the digestive apparatus finds that a part of its work has been done.

- **Cellulose:** Is the *most abundant* organic substance found in nature. This polysaccharide is found in *all* **plants,** forming the structure of its tissues: seeds, roots, stem, leaves, fruits, etc. In cereal seeds or grains, it is found in the covering skin, known as **bran.** In roots, leaves and fruits it is found intermingled with the vegetable structure.

Cellulose is also called **vegetable fiber.** It makes up the vegetable cells from which comes the name cellulose. Combined with lignin, it forms the wood of the trees. The molecules of cellulose are made up of a large chain of glucose molecules, but united in such a way that the digestive system cannot break them. Therefore, the cellulose cannot be absorbed and used for energy purposes.

- **Glycogen:** Is chemically similar to starch, but is produced by **animals** from the glucose which is freed by digestion and is absorbed and passed into the blood. Glycogen is stored in the liver and forms a **reserve** of energy which the body can use rapidly, being converted again into glucose, as it meets any energy

continues on page 41

Glucose
the universal fuel

Glucose with its chemical formula $C_6H_{12}O_6$ is the main fuel of the body. It may be said that from the viewpoint of energy, we are biologically, as **human beings,** a **motor** which **basically operates on glucose.**

Most of carbohydrates in food, (not fiber), **are transformed** into glucose within the digestive track, which passes to the blood and is carried to all cells of the body. But its main storage point is the **liver,** which operates as the **storehouse regulator.** The glucose is stored within this gland in the form of **glycogen**—reserve polysaccharides—which once more is converted into glucose when the body requires it. In this way the liver takes charge of maintaining a constant **glucose** level in the **blood:** approximately one gram for each liter of blood (**100 mg/100 ml**). A small quantity of glucose in the form of glycogen is also stored in the **muscle** cells, which is transformed again into glucose when any physical activity occurs.

When the level of glucose in the blood diminishes, and the reserves in the liver or the muscles (which last for only a few hours) are not able to raise it because they have been spent, then we have a **hypoglycemia** condition. If this happens suddenly, without giving the body time to find other sources of energy, notable symptoms result, such as dizziness, intense hunger, loss of strength, including the loss of consciousness and falling to the ground, a phenomenon which is known as lipothymia or fainting.

Glucose is transported by the blood to all the body cells. Thanks to the energy which it gives when burnt combined with the oxygen inside of the cells, glucose causes all the body to function. The **muscles** contract, heat is produced in the body, the **brain** carries on its functions, especially in the thought processes. To continue good operation, this marvelous organ needs to receive the supply of two substances without interruption: **glucose** and **oxygen.**

Each day our brain uses around 140 grams of glucose.

Glucose needs the action of the insulin hormone in order to be able to penetrate the cells, be burnt there, and produce energy. When there is insufficient insulin in the blood because the pancreas does not produce it, or because the cells cannot utilize that **insulin,** glucose accumulates in the blood, increasing its level there, instead of entering the cells to be used.

Once in the cells, the glucose needs Group **B vitamins** for the process of metabolism, that is, to be burned and produce energy. For this reason, when refined sugar is consumed (practically pure saccharose), the organism is forced to use its own vitamin B reserves to be able to metabolize that sugar, with the risk of using them up. **Refined sugar** is a very poor food: it only provides calories, but not the substances needed to be able to take advantage of them.

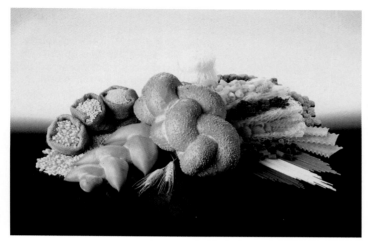

Bread and pasta provide the larger part of carbohydrates in the diet in the form of starch. Those that are prepared with refined flour as their base, with the typical white color, lack the vegetable fiber (bran) and vitamins B and E, that are found in wheat germ.

continues from page 39

demand (physical or mental effort, for example).

Glycogen is found in products originating in animals (liver and muscles) in small quantities, having practically **no food value.**

Objectives of a Healthful Diet when Dealing with Carbohydrates

According to the recommendation of WHO (World Health Organization)[1], a healthful diet should tend to:

1. *Increase* the consumption of *complex* carbohydrates (up to 70% of the ingested energy).

2. *Reduce* the consumption of refined *simple* carbohydrates (white sugar) as much as possible, until total exclusion is reached (lower limit -0%).

This means that the following foods should *be used* in *abundance:*

- **Grains/cereals** (wheat, barley, oats, rye, corn, rice, millet, etc.) They are the *main source* of *complex* carbohydrates (starch). According to the WHO, the abundant use of grains (especially oats) has beneficial results upon diabetes and other metabolic problems, and cuts down on the risk of cancer.

Cereals (grains) should once again become the *basis* of **human diet,** as it was throughout the past. The largest part of the energy that we need should come from them. This does not happen in the typical western diet which is based on meat, milk products, industrially produced canned and refined products, in which the proportion of energy coming from complex carbohydrates does not reach 50%. Experts in nutrition advise an abundant use of cereals, both at breakfast (in the form of bread, flakes, or cooked) as well as in the noon meal.

Furthermore, *authentic* **whole cereals** have the advantage of including the

1. WHO, Technical Report Series, No. 797, (*Diet, Nutrition, and the Prevention of Chronic Diseases*). Report of a WHO Study Group. Geneva, World Health Organization, 1990, pages 111, 113.

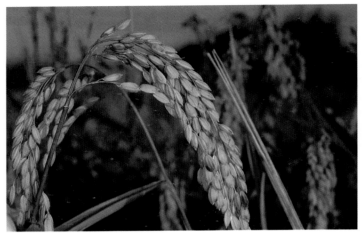

Rice, after wheat, is the most often used grain in the human diet. Whole rice should be used well cooked as semolina (groats), or in soup. In any other form it is difficult to chew its skin or bran. Rice contains a low quantity of sodium, and is therefore very good for those suffering hypertension and those who have heart problems.

grain's germ (rich in vitamins B and E, and in essential amino acids) and its covering of **bran** (rich in vegetable fiber).

- **Tubers** (yams or potatoes, for example) and **legumes,** also rich in complex **carbohydrates** (starch), aside from being a good source of **proteins,** have a great biological value.

- The typical *western diet,* based on meat, milk and its derivatives, is *very poor* in **vegetable fiber** (between three and ten grams daily). On the other hand, the diet based on **cereals, vegetables** and **fruit** generously provides the daily needs of vegetable fiber, according to the recommendations of the WHO.

The use of candy, pastries, sweets and drinks heavily laden with **sugar,** should be *reduced* to a *minimum.* According to the WHO, the use of refined (white) sugar, provides energy with no nutrients; that is, it supplies calories, but no minerals nor vitamins which are needed for this sugar to be metabolized. Therefore, it provokes an impoverishment in these substances.

On the other hand, unrefined sugar (brown), honey, and *above all,* the **natural** sugars found in **fruits,** are accompanied by few but useful amounts of **vitamins** and **minerals,** which allow good metabolic use.

Digestion and Use of Carbohydrates

Complex carbohydrates are turned into **glucose** in the intestine; but unlike that which takes place with simple sugars, the transformation into glucose happens slowly during digestion, and so its passage into the blood takes place *in steps.* On the other hand **simple sugars** (mono or disaccharides) enter the blood quickly, which *suddenly* raises the level of glucose. This provokes an intense response in the pancreas, which should rapidly secrete insulin in order to be able to metabolize all the glucose. As a result, a new lowering of glucose takes place in the blood (hypoglycemic crisis).

These *sudden* oscillations in the **glucose** level provoked by the eating of sweets, pastries, candies, etc. oblige the pancreas, and the body as a whole, to make great metabolic effort, thus opening the way to diseases such as **diabetes** or **arteriosclerosis.** This does not happen with complex

Vegetable Fiber

Cellulose or **vegetable fiber** is a special kind of **carbohydrate** which is **not absorbed** (does not go from the intestines to the blood), so that the body cannot use it as a source of energy. All that may be ingested is expelled with the feces. This fact led to its not being given any physiological importance in former decades. But now we understand the importance of that seemingly useless vegetable fiber: it acts as an authentic **broom** in the intestines, absorbing toxins and carrying out harmful substances such as biliary acids, the precursors of cholesterol.

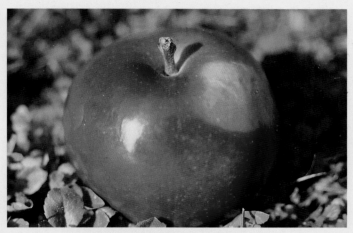
Apples are very rich in vegetable fiber.

Cellulose or vegetable fiber swells with water, increasing its volume several times. This gives consistency to the feces, and facilitates its transit through the colon until it is expelled through the rectum. When the diet contains little fiber because of the lack of fruit, whole grains and vegetables, the feces are hard, dry and concentrated, thus obliging the intestine to make enormous effort to eliminate them. This causes or worsens several problems, such as intestinal **diverticulum, hemorrhoids** and even **cancer** of the colon.

Cellulose (vegetable fiber) is **exclusive to the vegetable kingdom.** No animal food (meat, fish, milk or eggs) contains cellulose. Therefore, even though it does not provide energy, neither passes to the blood, it is an **indispensable component** of a healthy and balanced diet, since it **avoids constipation** (see page 168) and **lowers cholesterol.**

carbohydrates (starch from cereals, tubers, and legumes), which upon being digested and passed slowly to the blood, maintain a constant level of glucose for several hours, and allow for better functioning of the pancreas. This also explains why after having a sweet at breakfast, or enjoying a typical piece of toast covered with jelly, you are hungry again after a very short time, while if you have a breakfast based on whole cereals, you are not hungry the whole morning.

A diet based on cereals, fruits and vegetables perfectly satisfies all the needs for carbohydrates. Furthermore it provides the most healthful carbohydrates: starch and vegetable fiber.

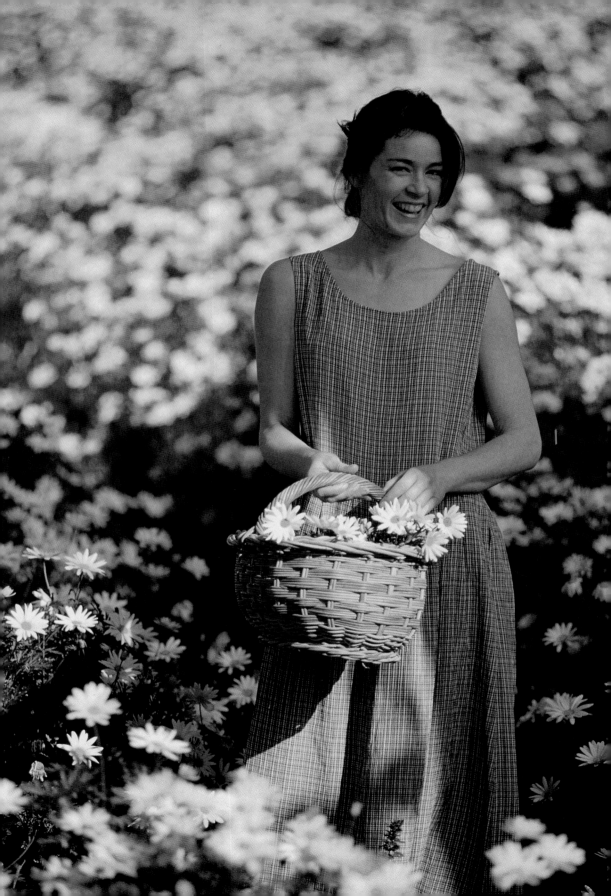

5

Fats

FATS OR lipids are chemical compounds which have in common the factor of being insoluble in water, and being formed basically of carbon, hydrogen and oxygen atoms. So they are formed from the same atoms as carbohydrates, but bonded in a different way.

Types of Fats

- **Simple lipids** or **neutral fats:** Are formed by the union of one glycerol molecule with another three fatty acids. This has led them to be called **triglycerides.**

- **Compound lipids** or **lipoids:** Into their structure, aside from the glycerol and fatty acids, enter other elements such as phosphorus, nitrogen and sulphur. Complex lipids are lecithin, cephalin, and sphingomyelin which fulfill important functions in the body, especially in the nerve tissues.

   Fatty acids are the main components of fats, to these they pass on their different

Don't ever repent of having eaten too little.

THOMAS JEFFERSON
USA President
from 1801 to 1809

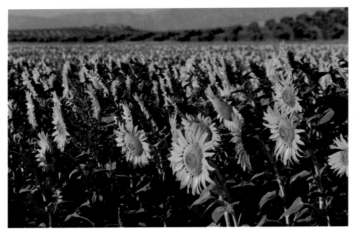

Sunflower seeds are rich in protein (27%), fats (49%) and minerals such as calcium (100 mg per 100 g), iron (7 mg per 100 g), and magnesium (420 mg per 100 g). From them a very smooth tasting oil is extracted, rich in unsaturated fatty acids (the most recommendable ones), such as linoleic acid.

tastes, textures and fluidity. From the chemical standpoint they consist of two types, very important to nutrition because their properties are very different:

- **Saturated fatty acids:** All their carbon atoms are united by simple links, which cause them to be saturated with hydrogen. Although all fats contain some saturated fatty acids, most of them come from **animal** foods. The palm nut and coconut are the exception between the plant foods as they contain more saturated than unsaturated fatty acids. The saturated fatty acids form **solid,** stable fats, reacting very little, and saturated in the fullest meaning of the word. Animals use these as a reserve substance. The abundant use of saturated fatty acids increases the **cholesterol** level in the blood, and is thought to increase the mortality caused by **cardiovascular diseases.**[1]

- **Unsaturated fatty acids:** They have one (monounsaturated), or more than one (polyunsaturated) double-bond between two or more of its carbon atoms. The most important sources of these fatty acids are from the **vegetable kingdom,** especially nuts, almonds and other oily dried products, and cereal germs.

The fat in **fish** also contains unsaturated fatty acids. They generally are in **liquid** form under room temperature (oils), and because all their carbon atoms are not saturated with hydrogen atoms, they retain a greater capacity to react with other substances and to be metabolized.

Oleic acid is a monounsaturated oily acid made up of 18 carbon atoms found especially in olive oil (76% of this is made up of glycerol and oleic acid), as well as in other seed oils.

Unsaturated fatty acids, such as the oleic found in olive oil, and especially polyunsaturated which are found in wheat germ, nuts, sunflower seeds, soybeans and grape seeds, are undoubtedly the most healthful. Furthermore, they have the interesting quality of *reducing* the production of **cholesterol** in the body.

---

1. WHO, Technical Report Series, No. 797, (*Diet, Nutrition, and the Prevention of Chronic Diseases*). Report of a WHO Study Group. Geneva, World Health Organization, 1990, pages 109, 110.

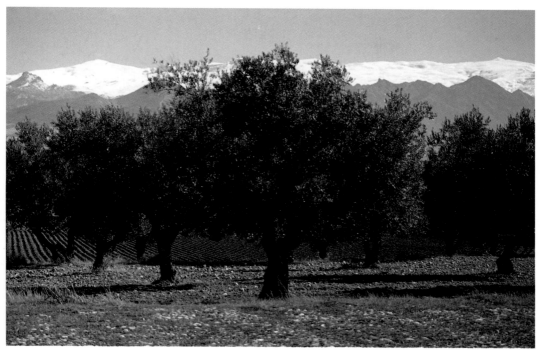

Olive oil is the king of oils, not only because of its exquisite taste, but because of its nutritive and medicinal qualities. It regulates cholesterol in the blood. It is used against constipation and in problems having to do with the gallbladder. Olives are rich in fats (36%) and also contain proteins (3%).

Digestion and the Use of Fats

Fats slow down the process of digestion, and thus give the sensation of a full stomach for a longer period of time. Fats are the most difficult nutrients for the digestive system to handle, and they overload the function of the two principal digestive glands: the liver and the pancreas. For this reason a diet that is very low in fats is recommended in the case of hepatitis or pancreatitis.

In the small intestine, because of the action of bile and lipase found in the pancreatic juice, fats are subdivided into their principal components: **glycerol** and **fatty acids.** In this way they cross the intestinal barrier and pass into the bloodstream. In the **liver** and in the **adipose tissues,** the body reunites the distinct elements which make up the fats, synthesizing its own, from the glycerol and the fatty acids which have been absorbed.

The body uses fats as combustible of high energy capability. One gram of fat produces 9 calories when it is burnt (metabolized), that is, over twice the same quantity of carbohydrates or proteins.

Daily Need of Fats

The recommendations of a study group of the WHO may be summarized into four points:

1. Reduce the total amount of fats which are included in the diet. The omnivorous diet typical of developed nations has an average of 45% of its calories in fats, which is an excessively high percentage. There are clear indications that the risk of certain types of cancer (for example the breast, the prostate and the colon) are directly related to the total amount of fats in the diet. *Not* more than *300 milligrams* daily of **cholesterol** should be included in the diet.

2. Reduce the use of saturated fatty acids until they are *completely eliminated.* These fatty acids have their source mainly in animals foods. As the ingestion of saturated fatty acids is reduced, there is a progressive reduction of deaths brought on by cardiovascular diseases. Since there is no known requirement for saturated fatty acids *per se* (except as a part of the total intake), the lower limit has been set by WHO at 0% of the total energy required.

3. Maintain a minimum consumption of polyunsaturated fatty acids which are found mainly in nuts, in seed oils (wheat germ, corn, soy beans, sunflower, etc.) and also in fish. These polyunsaturated fatty acids include those known as **essential fatty acids,** which are *indispensable* to the diet.

4. The monounsaturated fatty acids such as olive oil, should cover the difference between the total ingestion of fats and the sum of saturated and unsaturated fatty acids.

The vegetarian diet based on fruit, cereals, and vegetables completely satisfies these recommendations of the WHO because it is low in total fats, and rich in mono and

FATS
daily needs (WHO)

	% of total energy required	In a diet averaging 2,000 calories this is equivalent to:	
Total fats			
Lower limit	15 %	300 calories	33 grams
Upper limit	30 %	600 calories	67 grams
Respect different specific types of fats			
Saturated fatty acids			
Lower limit	0 %	0 calories	0 grams
Upper limit	10 %	200 calories	22 grams
Polynsaturated fatty acids			
Lower limit	3 %	60 calories	7 grams
Upper limit	7 %	140 calories	16 grams

polyunsaturated fats. This is not the case in a diet based on meat and its derivatives, which contain an excess of fats (up to 45% of the total calories) and an excess of saturated fatty acids of animal origin.

Cholesterol

Cholesterol is a complex lipid (a kind of fat) of the group of sterols which are found *exclusively* in foods originating from **animals,** and which our body furthermore produces in the liver. Its function in the body is to provide raw material for the synthesizing of sexual hormones, among others, of the biliary salts and cellular membranes.

Although it is an indispensable substance of life, when its level increases within the blood, it tends to be deposited in the walls of the arteries, weakening them and narrowing their passageway, which is known as **arteriosclerosis.** For this reason, a high level of cholesterol tends to increase the risk of a myocardial attack, arterial thrombosis and a lack of blood supply to the extremities.

Cholesterol circulates throughout the blood connected to substances known as **lipoproteins.** According to the type of lipoprotein connected to the cholesterol, it has different names, and their effects are distinct:

LDL Cholesterol

It is the cholesterol which circulates through the blood united to **low density lipoproteins** (LDL). It represents approximately **75%** of the total blood cholesterol. The LDL cholesterol favors the development of arteriosclerosis. It is called the **"bad** or harmful **cholesterol."**

HDL Cholesterol

It circulates with the **high-density lipoproteins** (HDL). It has been shown recently that this kind of cholesterol, known commonly as **"good cholesterol"** is a preventive of arteriosclerosis. The more there is in the blood level, the better.

CHOLESTEROL
in some foods

Food	Content in miligrams for each 100 grams	Quantity of food in grams which provides the maximun 300 mg allowed daily
Brains	2,195	14
Egg yolk	1,281	23
Beef liver	309	97
Meat fat	300	100
Butter	219	137
Gruyere cheese	110	273
Lobsters	95	316
Veal loin	83	361
Pork chops	72	417
Pork sausage	68	441
Chicken, lamb	68	441
Cod fish	55	545
Oysters	50	600
Whole milk	13.6	2,206
Whole yogurt	12.7	2,362
Low fat milk	7.5	4,000
Skimmed milk	2	15,000
Fruit	0	–
Cereals	0	–
Vegetables	0	–

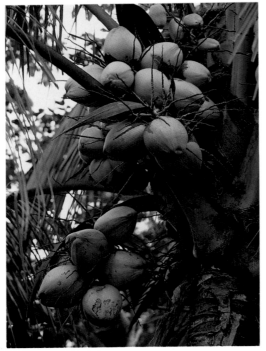

The oil obtained from coconuts, different from other vegetable oils, has a large amount of saturated fatty acids. It is used in margarine and in ice cream, and should not be used excessively. On the other hand, water from the young coconut is a refreshing drink and is very healthful.

From the table at the page 38, it can be determined that olive oil, although it cuts down very little on the total cholesterol, exercises a protective effect on the formation of arteriosclerosis as it increases the "good cholesterol" carried by the high density lipoproteins (HDL cholesterol).

The **oils** of seeds, rich in polyunsaturated fatty acids, reduce the total cholesterol, but also the protective HDL, so that its total effect on the reduction of the risk of arteriosclerosis, though important, is incomplete. Taking all this into consideration, a good recommendation is to use olive oil together with seed oils, not mixing them, but alternating their use.

Fish, especially the fatty type, contain polyunsaturated fatty acids which lower the cholesterol level. But it should be remembered that because fish belongs to the animal kingdom, it also contains cholesterol which is absorbed and passed to the blood. Because of this, the total effect of fish upon blood cholesterol, and their protective action upon arteriosclerosis, is not as notable as might be expected.

continues on page 52

FATTY ACIDS: effect on CHOLESTEROL

Type of Fatty Acids	Source	Effect Upon Cholesterol	
		LDL	HDL
Saturated	Animal fat	Increase	Increase
Monounsaturated	Olive oil, avocado	Neutral or decrease	Neutral or slight increase
Polyunsaturated	Seed oils, fish	Decrease	Decrease

Suggestions for the Reduction of Cholesterol Levels

- **Decrease** the use of **meat,** especially beef and pork, as well as viscera, sausages, etc.
- Learn to cook without egg yolks.
- Do not eat more than **three** whole **eggs per week.** There is no limit to egg whites (cholesterol is found only in the yolk).
- Preferably use low fat or **fat free** milk and dairy products, especially avoiding cream, butter and fatty cheeses.
- **Reduce** the use of commercial **sweets,** pastries, and desserts containing animal fats.
- **Increase** the use of vegetable **fiber** (whole grains, fruits, especially apples, and vegetables), which absorb the biliary salts needed for the formation of cholesterol in the intestines.
- Use **olive oil,** alternating with **seed oils** (corn, wheat germ, sunflower, grape seeds etc.)
- **Avoid** nervous **tension** and **stress.**
- Perform **physical exercise** daily (for at least one half hour).
- Keep your weight down.

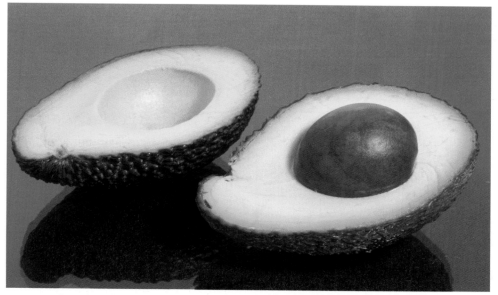

In spite of its heavy fat content (23.5%), avocados lower the level of cholesterol in the blood because of its large content of polyunsaturated fatty acids, especially linoleic acid.

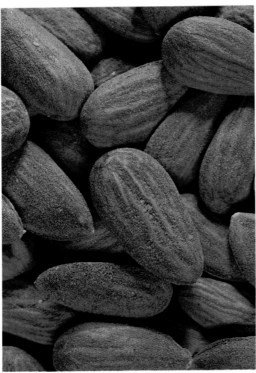

Linoleic Acid
in some foods

Food	Content in grams for each 100 grams	Quantity of food in g providing the recommended daily allowance (6 g)
Nut	32	19
Dry soybeans	11	55
Almonds	10	60
Avocado	1.8	333
Eggs	1.2	500
Milk	0.6	1,000
Beef	0.2	3,000
Salmon	0.08	7,500

Almonds are one of the vegetable products with the largest concentration of proteins (18.3%) and fats (54%), as well as vitamins and minerals. Because of their richness in polyunsaturated fatty acids, they lower the cholesterol level in the blood.

continues from page 50

Linoleic Acid
functions

- Body growth
- Building of nerve tissue
- Formation and renewal of the skin and its annexes (hair, nails, etc.)
- Synthesis of the prostaglandines
- Lowers blood cholesterol and heart attack risk

Essential fatty acids

They are the polyunsaturated fatty acids which our bodies are not capable of synthesizing, and which we must continually ingest throughout life. For this reason they have been called in the past **vitamin F** (from fat), though they actually are not vitamins.

Linoleic acid and **linolenic acid** are found principally in grain germs (wheat, corn, oats, etc.) and in nuts (walnuts, almonds, hazel nuts, etc.) Animal foods also contain these acids, although in a proportion ten times smaller and always accompanied by saturated fatty acids and cholesterol harmful to health.

Fats
norms for their culinary use

1. **Limit the use** of foods high in fats. Both carbohydrates and proteins are digested more slowly when they have been cooked in fats.

2. Use fats obtained from **vegetables** (olive or seed oil) instead of animal fats (butter, bacon, or lard).

3. **Avoid fried foods,** especially when dealing with animal products (meat and fish). Fats, especially the animal fats, decompose at high temperatures, as happens during the frying process. Thus, irritating substances are formed such as acrolein, which is highly indigestible, producing a feeling of heaviness in the stomach, and intestinal discomfort. Animal fats produce carcinogenic substances at fairly low temperatures but vegetable oils must get to the smoking point to produce such.

   If you must fry, it is preferable to use vegetable products, at not excessively high temperatures, changing the oil each time. **Olive oil** is the most stable at high temperatures, thus being more adequate for frying. Seed oils oxidize more easily and are less appropriate for frying.

4. **Do not** use **more than two foods rich in fats** in one meal (for example, avocados, mayonnaise, ice cream, or cream).

5. Control the use of **hidden fats** which often accompany prepared or canned foods, such as french fries, chocolate, crackers, pastries or preserves.

Deficits of these essential fatty acids are revealed in growth retardation, dryness of the skin, dermatitis, and nerve and genital diseases.

The WHO recommends the ingestion of polyunsaturated fatty acids to range between **3%** and **7%** of the total calories in the diet. For a diet averaging 2,000 calories this represents between 7 and 16 grams of **polyunsaturated fatty acids** per day, of which at least 6 grams should be **linoleic acid.** Nevertheless, it is advisable to surpass this lower limit and reach up to 12 grams per day of linoleic acid (6% of the energy for a 2,000 calories diet).

To assure the lower limit of linoleic acid, the vegetarian diet is the surest, for it is enough, for example, to eat 60 grams of almonds each day. Cow milk is lacking in linoleic acid, therefore it is recommended that seed oils, which are rich in this acid, be added to the dietary preparations aimed at feeding little children.

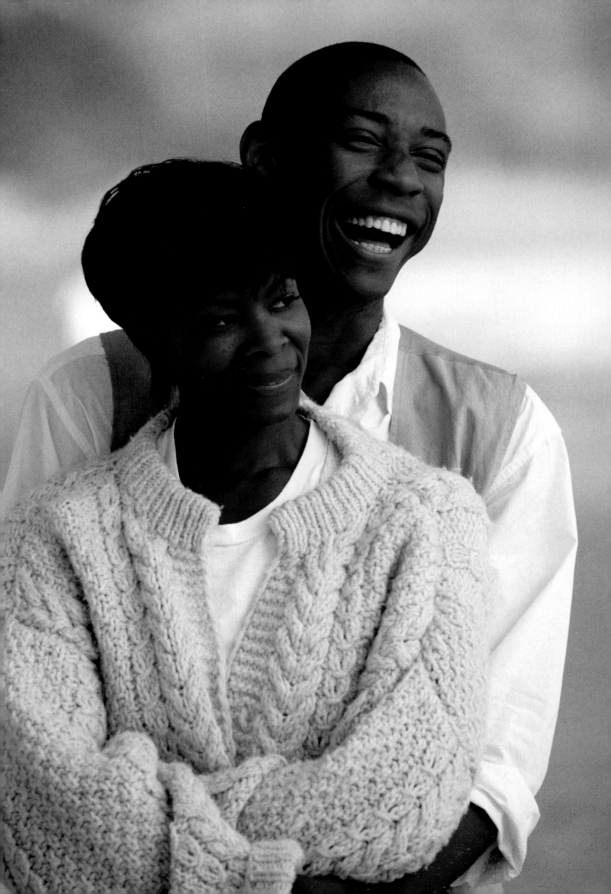

6

Proteins

WHERE DO you get your proteins? Do you eat sufficient proteins? These are the two questions which a vegetarian often has to hear. There is a great interest in proteins in the diet. And this is not in vain, for these nutrients present two peculiar characteristics:

- **They form the basis** of the structure of **the body,** being the most important component of muscles, blood, skin and all the internal organs. Bones are formed of collagen proteins, upon which calcium and other minerals are based. Around 17% of our body weight is made up of proteins, that is, from 10 to 12 kilos for a normal adult.

- **They are not stored** in the organism to form an alimentary reserve, different from what happens with carbohydrate or fats. For this reason it is necessary to ingest them constantly throughout life.

continues on page 57

**Others live to eat,
but I eat to live.**

SOCRATES
Greek philosopher,
5th century B.C.

Proteins in some foods

Food	Content in grams per 100 grams	Quantity of food in g providing the recommended daily allowance (52.5 g)*	Food	Content in grams per 100 grams	Quantity of food in g providing the recommended daily allowance (52.5 g)*
Soybeans	37	142	Tomatoes	1.2	4,375
Raw lentils	28	188	Onions	1.16	4,526
Fresh peanuts	26	202	Cucumbers	0.7	7,500
Sunflower seed	23	228	Coconut (dry pulp)	3.3	1,591
Almonds	20	263	Dry figs	3.1	1,694
Raw chick peas	19	276	Avocados	2	2,625
Pine nuts	12	438	Cherries	1.2	4,375
Soy sprouts	3	1,750	Oranges	0.9	5,833
Oats	17	309	Olives	0.8	6,563
Whole bread	14	375	Fresh tuna	23	2,536
Raw macaroni	13	404	Chicken	21	250
Wheat	10.4	505	Veal	20	263
White bread	10.3	510	Fresh hake	19	276
Corn	9	583	Pork	18.3	287
Rice	7	750	Fresh cod	18	292
Fresh peas	5	1,050	Lamb chops	15	350
Alfalfa	4	1,313	Cottage cheese	13.7	383
Artichokes	3	1,750	Eggs	13	404
Mushrooms	2.09	2,512	Yogurt	3.5	1,500
Potatoes	2.07	2,536	Milk	3.3	1,591

* The calculations are based on a daily allowance of 0.75 g of proteins per kg of weight (for male adults, 70 kilos = 154 lb), as recommended by the WHO (0.75 g/kg x 70 kg = 52.5 g of proteins).

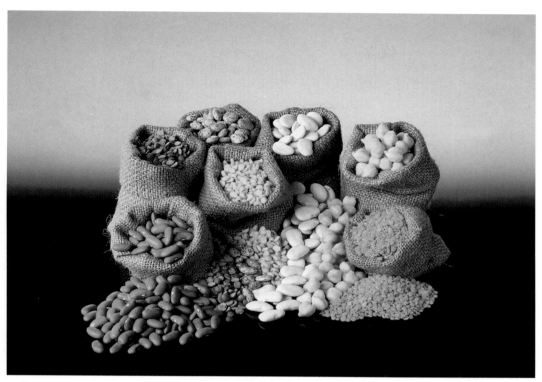

Legumes make up a large family of plants which includes beans and peas. The percentage of protein and iron in these is equal or superior to that found in meat. They are a basic element in the Mediterranean diet. Soybeans are the legume that has the most complete protein.

continues from page 55

Chemical Composition

Each protein is made up of a variable number of **amino acids** (from just a few up to the thousands) united in a long chain. These amino acids, in their turn, are formed by carbon, oxygen and hydrogen atoms (like carbohydrates and fats). In addition, they contain a fourth element characteristic of proteins: **nitrogen.**

Amino acids are like bricks used to construct a protein building. The nature and characteristic of each protein depends on the type of amino acids which form it, and above all, on the order in which they form the chain.

Digestion and the Use of Proteins

Upon arrival in the stomach, the proteins are attacked by **pepsin,** an enzyme which initiates the task of breaking down the union which exists among the amino acids. Later on, in the small intestine, **trypsin** from the pancreatic juice and other enzymes complete the task of separating the amino acids that made up the protein.

PROTEINS
daily needs according to age[*]

Age	Grams
0-1 years	13-14
1-3 years	16
4-6 years	24
7-10 years	28
Males 11-24 years	45-58
Males adults	63
Females 11-24 years	46
Females adults	50
Pregnant women	60
Lactating women	65

* Recommended Dietary Allowances (revised 1989), according to the US Food and Nutrition Board, National Academy of Sciences—National Research Council.

Essential Amino Acids

As surprising as it may appear, all proteins in nature are basically formed of not many more than 20 different kinds of amino acids. Combining them in various forms, in number and order, makes it possible to have the great variety of proteins which make up living beings.

Man and animals are able to transform some amino acids into others (a process which takes place in the liver) to synthesize its own proteins, but with certain limitations. There are **eight amino acids** (**10** in children), which are called **essential,** which should always be included in the diet, because they cannot be made by the organism. A varied **vegetarian diet** provides **all** of the essential amino acids, and in the necessary proportion.

Actually, amino acids of **all** the **proteins** ultimately come from **plants,** for they are the only ones capable of taking advantage of the nitrogen in the atmosphere or in the soil

The amino acids which are thus freed are absorbed into the small intestine, and pass to the blood from which they are distributed to all the body cells. These cells, especially those of the **liver,** use the amino acids to synthesize the body proteins, assembling them in a new order and proportion specific to each living being. Amino acids that are left over, if there are any, may be metabolized to be converted into energy, or may be transformed into fats or glucose.

Essential Amino Acids

Adults	Children
Isoleucine	Isoleucine
Leucine	Leucine
Lysine	Lysine
Methionine	Methionine
Phenylalanine	Phenylalanine
Threonine	Threonine
Tryptophane	Tryptophane
Valine	Valine
	Histidine
	Arginine

Some Situations in Which an Increased Consumption of Proteins Is Recommended

- Times of **growth** (children and adolescents)
- **Pregnancy** and **lactation**
- **Convalescence** from infectious diseases or from surgery
- In cases of persistent excessive **perspiration**
- Exposure to **extreme temperatures,** cold and heat
- Persistent conditions of **nervous tension**

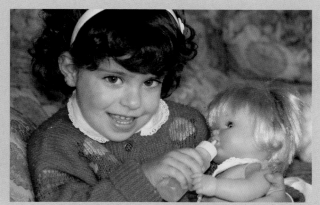

In relation to their weight, children need twice the amount of proteins as adults.

to produce amino acids and proteins. Beings from the animal kingdom are not able to produce organic substances beginning with the chemical elements that compose them, and all they can do is feed upon plants or other animals that have eaten vegetables. It is only in this way that they may obtain the amino acids needed to build their own proteins.

The Need for Proteins

The amount of proteins found in the regular diet in developed countries is probably in excess of actual needs. This is a fact which is accepted by all nutritional experts after so many years in which there was an insistence that more proteins should be eaten. At present the WHO recommends a daily intake of **0.75 grams** of proteins **per kilo** of weight, which represents 52.5 grams per day for a man weighing 70 kilos (154 lb). This is equivalent to the recommended daily allowance of 63 grams for a male adult weighting 79 kg (174 lb) [0.80 grams per kilo of weight], as stated by the US National Research Council.

The WHO further recommends that **calories** proceeding from proteins vary between **10%** and **15%** of the total calories in the diet. For a diet of 2,500 calories per day, this would mean between 62 and 93 grams per day, and for a diet of 2,000 calories, between 50 and 75 grams.

A study of the table of protein content of foods reveals that it is not difficult to obtain these daily grams of proteins. Let's look at one example:

Proteins and Physical Exercise

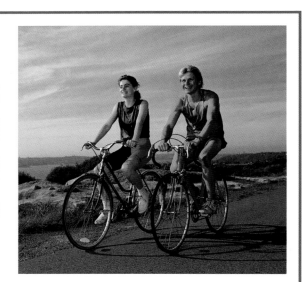

Although there appears to be a contradiction, **intense physical activity does not imply an increased need for proteins***. This has been demonstrated in numerous studies of athletes, though many trainers continue to recommend that athletes consume diets that have a high protein content. What athletes really need is a larger amount of complex carbohydrates (whole cereals).

Only those practicing body building leading to an abnormal development of their muscles, which is certainly not recommended for health, need to increase their use of proteins.

* GRANDE COVIÁN, F. *Nutrition and Health.* Madrid, Today's Issues Publications, 1990, page 127.

Food	Grams of protein
Lentils (2 ounces)	14
Sunflower seeds (52 gramos)	12
Crema de cacahuete (2 cucharadas)	8
Pan integral de trigo o cebada (2 rebanadas)	5
Germen de trigo (2 cucharadas)	3
Guisantes (60 gramos)	12
Total	**54**

Quality and Source of Proteins

All living organisms, whether plant or animal, contain proteins. Actually, **animal proteins** also **come from plants,** for as we have noted, only these are able to use the atmospheric or mineral nitrogen to form amino acids. Animals take advantage of the property of plants and use the amino acids that only they are able to synthesize.

Proteins found in fruits, cereals and different vegetables contain the 20 amino acids needed for human nutrition, including the essential ones. Animal proteins are formed beginning with the plant amino acids. The

A varied and balanced vegetarian diet, especially if it is combined with milk and/or eggs, is highly satisfactory for the development of a child.

difference between plant and animal proteins lies only in the proportion of amino acids which they contain, and in their order. Animal proteins have a larger proportion of essential amino acids for our nutrition; that is, they are more concentrated.

As far as the liver is concerned, when it is manufacturing the proteins of our bodies, it makes no difference whether a certain amino acid comes from a plant, or from an animal which consumed plants. What is important is that it is available in the blood.

What we need are amino acids, not specific proteins, as for example those found in meat. All experts agree, and experience has demonstrated, that **meat is not indispensable** in human diet for the enjoyment of **good health.** This is a fairly recent concept in the science of nutrition. Up to a few decades ago, it was thought that people should eat proteins that were more similar to their own. And an unjustified superiority was given to animal proteins over plant proteins, which were apparently less valued.

Variety Is the Key

Proteins which have their source in animals (meat, fish, milk products and eggs) have been called **complete** because they contain all the amino acids that our body needs, and in an optimal proportion.

Proteins which have their source in vegetables are called **incomplete** (except soybeans) because one or several of their amino acids are not in the correct proportion that our body needs. If an experimental animal is fed only on wheat, even though it may be whole, it does not grow enough. But if this diet is complemented with a legume (lentils, for example) there is normal growth.

Another example: **legumes** are *low* in two essential amino acids: **methionine** and **tryptophane.** On the other hand **cereals,** or **milk,** are *rich* in these. Therefore, with a mixture of legumes with cereals our body gets all of the needed amino acids, and will be able to produce good and sufficient quality proteins.

Combinations Which Provide Proteins of Good Quality

Milk or Milk Products with Cereals

✓ Dried cereal with milk

✓ Oat flakes or oat flakes with other cereals cooked in milk

✓ Rice with cottage cheese

✓ Bread and cottage cheese

Cereals with Legumes

✓ Rice with lentils (peas)

✓ Rice with sweet peas

✓ Wheat or oat flakes with chick peas

✓ Rice and beans

Legumes with Vegetables

✓ Green beans and tomatoes

✓ Vegetable soup with beans

✓ Lentils with potatoes

Cereals with Vegetables

✓ Corn with green beans

✓ Rice with vegetables (green peppers, carrots, onions, etc.)

Today we know that, thanks to the phenomenon of supplementation, the quality of vegetable protein increases when these are combined among themselves, or are combined with milk and/or eggs. In this way, the vegetable proteins provide all the essential amino acids and reach a biological value comparable to meat, without any of its side effects.

Here we arrive at a fundamental concept: Vegetable proteins, in general, are incomplete by themselves. But when they are combined, including various vegetables in the same meal, one **complements** the other, and among all together, the body receives the needed amino acids. This interesting phenomenon is known as **supplementation.** Although it is not necessary to eat a combination of grain and legume at each meal—as long as both are eaten within the space of 2-3 meals or during the day.

When the diet has proteins derived from different sources, and above all, if they are eaten at the same meal, the body is able to obtain sufficient amino acids to form the proteins that it needs. Combining the various types of vegetables is easy and it tastes good. Several examples of good combinations have been given in the chart on this page.

Milk or eggs, because they contain the most complete and digestible proteins, complement any vegetable food perfectly. For that reason, the ovolactovegetarian diet is very satisfactory, and those who follow it run no risk of following a deficient diet. It is sufficient to use milk or eggs with cereals, legumes and other vegetables, to get all the needed amino acids. So, **ovolactovegetari-**

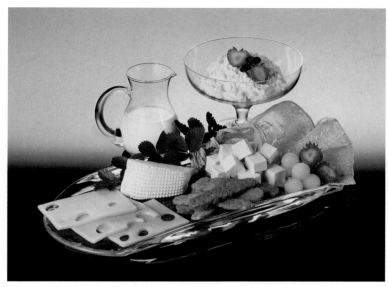

The proteins of milk and its derivatives are complete in themselves, so that with a lactovegetarian diet there is no danger of any nutritional deficiency. It must be remembered that milk products have the problem of being rich in saturated fats and cholesterol. For this reason adults, should use them in their low-fat form.

ans or **lactovegetarians,** including children, do not have to worry a great deal about proteins.

Those who follow a **strict vegetarian diet** may equally be well nourished, and obtain proteins of as high a quality as meat, milk, eggs or fish. This is recognized by such noted researchers as Miguel Aguilar,[1] of the Superior Council of Scientific Research of Spain, and Doctor Joan Sabaté,[2] of Loma Linda University (USA) This requires a certain degree of attention and knowledge of nutritional science, so that there will be an adequate combination of various vegetables.

Children and **pregnant women** need a larger share and a better quality of protein. Though it is possible that they may follow a strict vegetarian diet without any ill effects, and experience has demonstrated this, the various foods must be selected and carefully combined. Not all individuals have the knowledge or the time needed for this. Therefore, as a general recommendation, we prefer to counsel children and pregnant women who are vegetarians to complement their diet with milk products and eggs. In this way, they may be sure that their diet is complete and healthful.

The vegetarian diet based on fruits, cereals and vegetables is more healthy than the omnivorous (the diet of those who eat everything), but it requires greater attention and knowledge of nutrition, as well as a progressive application (pages 139, 171).

1. AGUILAR, M. *La dieta vegetariana.* Madrid, Ediciones Temas de Hoy, 1990, page 251.
2. SABATÉ, J. *Growth in vegetarian children* [El crecimiento en los niños vegetarianos]. Doctoral Thesis, University of Loma Linda (California, USA), 1988.

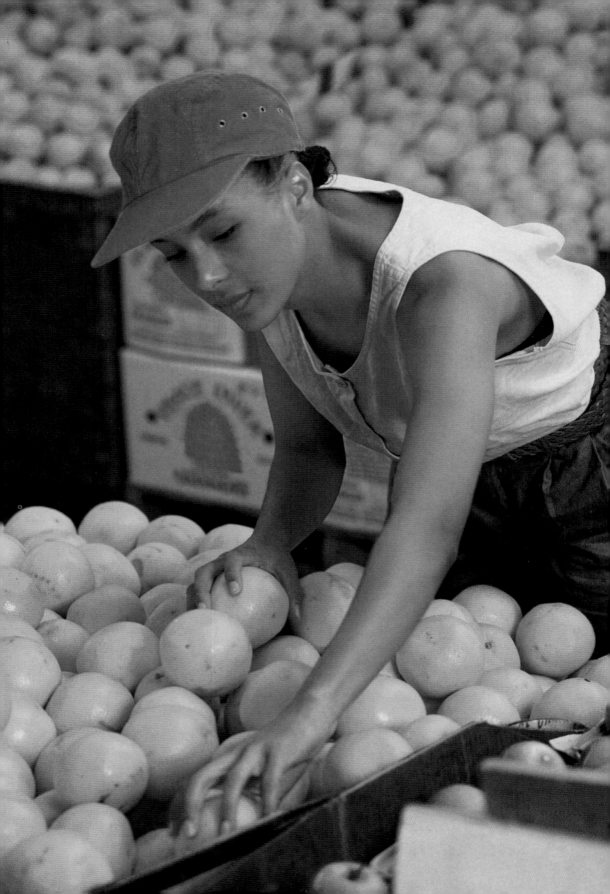

7

Vitamins

V ITAMINS are organic substances which play important functions in our body. It needs vitamins in very small quantities, and cannot produce them by itself, so vitamins must be provided by foods.

Knowledge concerning vitamins is fairly recent. Actually all of them were discovered during the twentieth century. Nevertheless, it was already known that when experimental animals were fed a diet containing pure carbohydrates, fats, and proteins, animals ceased to grow, became ill and finally died.

The dream of some scientist of being able to feed themselves with a chemically pure diet, creating synthetic foods, vanished. Animals and men need more than carbohydrates, fats and proteins, as abundant as they may be. There should be, therefore, some substances in the foods in their natur-

All that is necessary has been created.

<small>PHILOSOPHICAL PRINCIPLE</small>

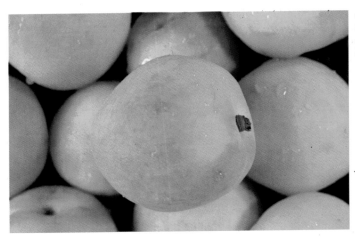

Apricots are one of the richest fruits in vitamin A, present in the form of carotene, its provitamin.

al state that are indispensable to life. In 1912 the Polish biochemist **Casimir Funk** called these substances the "amines of life" or vitamins.

During the following decades, scientists dedicated themselves to an intense search for these precious substances which were so indispensable to life. As they were discovered, they were identified with a letter from the alphabet. New substances have been found up to the present time, especially in the vegetable kingdom, which fulfill functions in the body that cannot be substituted. This is the case with folic acid, which is found in green vegetables and nuts, and the polyunsaturated acids of vegetable oils (see page 52).

Source of Vitamins

Vitamins are primarily produced within the vegetable kingdom, whether it be in the higher level of plants, mushrooms or bacteria. In some cases animals may transform them and store them as it happens, for example, with vitamins A and D, which plants produce as provitamins, and which are stored in the liver of fish and mammals as vitamins. Nevertheless the **basic source** of vitamins are **vegetable** foods. Meat and fish, for example, are very deficient in vitamin C.

Vitamin A

Vitamin A is found in the colored vegetables (carrots, tomatoes, greens, etc.) in the form of *provitamin,* known as **beta-carotene,** that our body transforms into true vitamin A (**retinol**), according to the body needs. Since the intestinal absorption of carotenes is not as easy as vitamin A which comes from animals, it is calculated that we need six times more vegetable carotene than animal retinol. Even so the normal vegetarian diet provides more than enough vitamin A. This does not happen in the case of animal foods, in which, excepting animal livers, certain fish, or milk derivatives, it is very low. Lean meat is very poor in vitamin A.

According to the WHO, vitamin A is one of the ***most scarce*** vitamins in certain areas of the world.

Functions

- Formation of the **visual pigments** in the retina. The lack of vitamin A impedes seeing in poor light (night blindness).

- Forming and maintaining the **cells** which **cover** the skin, eyes, mouth and internal organs. When there is a lack of vitamin A, the **skin,** and especially the **membrane** which covers the eye, are weakened and dry up. When this deficit happens, serious blindness is a result. Many cases of blindness caused by the lack of vitamin A take place among the children of the third world.

- It reduces the risks of the formation of cancerous tumors in the organs of our body, due to its strong **antioxidant** action. This effect is produced in its form of vegetable provitamin (carotene). It has been proven that smokers who eat many vegetables, especially carrots, suffer less lung cancer than smokers that eat few. Cancer risk is lower in those who eat foods containing this vitamin and even more so in those eating fresh fruits and vegetables than in those who just take the vitamin in pill form.

Excess is Also Dangerous

Just as it happens with another fat-soluble vitamin, vitamin D, an excess of vitamin A in its final state (retinol), as is found in animals, is toxic to man. For this reason, it is recommended that hunters in the Arctic not eat fox or polar bear livers, which accumulate large quantities of vitamin A. In the same way, pharmaceutical preparations of vitamin A should contain a warning of the risk involved in taking more than the advised dosage. Poisoning symptoms, known clinically as **hypervitaminosis A,** are: fatigue,

Vitamin A
in some foods

Food	Content in of RE* per 100 grams	Quantity of food in g providing the recommended daily allowance (1000 RE)
Alfalfa	16,000	6
Carrots	2,813	36
Spinach	672	149
Beets	610	164
Parsley	520	192
Mango	389	257
Fresh apricots	261	383
Persimmons	217	461
Papaya	175	571
Tomatoes	64	1,563
Bell peppers	63	1,587
Melons	3	33,333
Turnip	0	–
Veal liver	4,427	23
Butter	754	133
Tuna	655	153
Milk	31	3,226
Cod fish	12	8,333
Veal	0	–

* Retinol Equivalent (RE) of vitamin A = **1 µg** of retinol (animal vitamin A) = **6 µg** of **beta-carotene** (vegetable provitamin A). This is because the beta-carotene is less absorbed than retinol.

Vitamin A
daily needs

Children	400 - 700 RE
Males adults	1,000 RE
Females adults	800 RE
Pregnant	800 RE
Lactating	1,300 RE

Vitamin B₁
in some foods

Food	Conten in miligrams per 100 grams	Quantity of food in g providing the recommended daily allowance (1.5 mg)
Brewer's yeast	12	13
Wheat germ	1.9	79
Pine nuts	1.2	125
Fresh soybeans	0.9	167
Garbanzos	0.48	313
Whole wheat	0.45	333
Sweet peas	0.27	556
Almond	0.21	714
Lentils	0.17	882
Cherimoya	0.1	1,500
Oranges	0.09	1,667
Artichokes	0.07	2,143
Figs	0.06	2,500
Blackberries	0.03	5,000
Pork	0.8	188
Fresh salmon	0.23	652
Veal liver	0.19	789
Lamb chops	0.1	1,500
Veal	0.08	1,875
Egg yolk	0.17	882
Milk	0.04	3,947

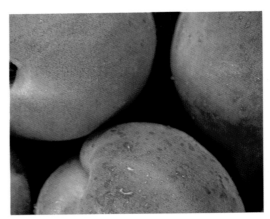

Among fresh fruits, peaches are one of the richest in vitamin B₂.

nervousness, pain in the bones, decalcification, headaches, and dizziness.

A **vegetarian diet** satisfactorily covers the needs for vitamin A, in the form of carotene. Aside from possessing interesting preventive effects against cancer, with carotene (vegetable provitamin A) there is no risk of overdosage, since the body produces only the vitamin A that it needs.

Vitamin B₁ (Thiamin)

At the beginning of this century, vitamin B₁ or thiamin was discovered in whole rice, when it was observed that this food was able to cure beriberi.

Vitamin B₁
daily needs

Children . . . . 0.7 - 1 mg
Male adults . . . . 1.5 mg
Female Adults . . . . 1.1 mg
Pregnant . . . . 1.5 mg
Lactating . . . . 1.6 mg

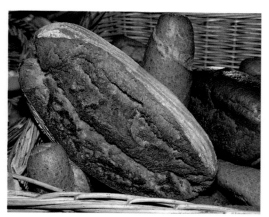

Bread baked with authentic whole wheat flour, also includes wheat germ, very rich in vitamins B₁, B₂, B₆, and E, as well as essential amino acids. This is not the case with some flours which are made simply by mixing white flour with bran.

Vitamin B₂ in some foods		
Food	Content in miligrams per 100 grams	Quantity of food in g providing the recommended daily allowed (1.7 mg)
Brewer´s yeast	3.8	45
Almendras	0.8	213
Wheat germ	0.5	340
mushrooms	0.45	378
Algae	0.34	500
Walnuts	0.15	1,133
Avocados	0.12	1,417
Peaches	0.04	4,250
Eggs	0.5	340
Veal	0.28	607
Fresh tuna	0.25	680
Ham	0.23	739
Milk	0.16	1,049
Chicken	0.14	1,214

Functions

- It intervenes in the **metabolism** of **carbohydrates,** facilitating the chemical reaction through which its final product, **glucose,** is transformed into energy.
- Is an essential factor in the function of the **nervous system.** Its absence results in irritability and nervous imbalance.

A lack of vitamin B₁ causes **beriberi,** a disease which fortunately has become rare in the world. Vitamin B₁ is widely found throughout nature, *all* **fruits, cereals** (especially the whole grain ones) and **vegetables**

Vitamin B₂ daily needs	
Children.	0.8 - 1.2 mg
Male adults	1.7 mg
Female adults	1.3 mg
Pregnant	1.6 mg
Lactating	1.8 mg

have it. White sugar (not honey or molasses), and refined white flour (not the whole flour) are poor in vitamin B₁. A diet based on fruit, cereals and vegetables provides more than enough to meet the needs for this vitamin.

Vitamin B₂ (Riboflavin)

Functions

It favors body **growth,** catalyzing the chemical reactions needed for taking advantage of carbohydrates and proteins. Its lack provokes a slowing down in growth, as well

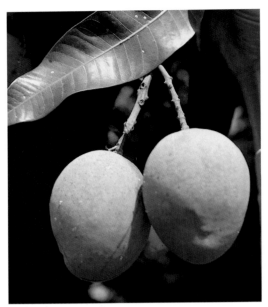

Mango is a tropical fruit with an exquisite taste and a fair content of vitamin A.

Food	Content in miligrams per 100 grams	Quantity of food in g providing the recommended daily allowance (2 mg)
Wheat germ	1.3	154
Bananas	0.58	345
Nuts	0.56	357
brown rice	0.51	392
Avocado	0.5	400
Soybeans	0.38	526
Bell peppers	0.25	800
Polished rice	0.15	1,333
White flour	0.04	5,000
White sugar	0	–
Lean pork	0.51	392
lean veal	0.43	465
Mackerel	0.4	500
Sardines	0.12	1,667

Vitamin B$_6$
in some foods

as alterations in the skin and the retina (sight deficiency).

Vitamin B$_2$ is widely distributed among all plant foods especially in nuts and dried fruits, as well as grain germs. The spirula algae and brewer's yeast are some of the most concentrated sources of vitamin B$_2$.

Vitamin B$_6$ (Pyridoxine)

Functions

It regulates the **metabolism** of **proteins,** especially in the nerve tissues, the liver, and the skin. It contributes to the formation of **red cells** in the blood.

Its lack is manifested in symptoms of fatigue, nervousness, anemia and changes in the skin.

Vitamin B$_6$
daily needs

Children	1 - 1.4 mg
Male adults.	2 mg
Female adults	1.6 mg
Pregnant.	2.2 mg
Lactating	2.1 mg

Vitamin B12
in some foods

Food	Content in micrograms (µg) per 100 grams	Quantity of food in g providing the recommended daily allowance (2 µg)
Spirula*	100	2
Veal liver	47	4
Red herring	14	14
Lamb	2.6	77
Beef	2.4	83
Canned tuna	2.2	91
Cheese	1.3	154
Eggs	1	200
Cottage cheese	0.5	400
Chicken	0.37	541
Yogurt	0.37	541
Milk	0.36	560

* According to some researchers, our bodies handly take advantage of the vitamin B12 found in the spirula algae.

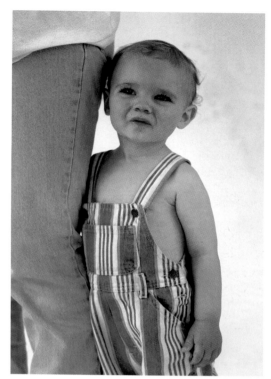

There is no risk of a lack of vitamin B12 in a ovolactovegetarian diet. Strict vegetarians may need supplements of vitamin B12, especially children.

Vitamin B12
daily needs

Children	0.7 - 1.4 µg
Male adults	2 µg
Female adults	2 µg
Pregnant.	2.2 µg
Lactating.	2.6 µg

Vitamin B6 is found in **cereals,** especially the **whole grain** ones, fruits and vegetables, as well as in milk, eggs, and meat. Avocados, bananas, nuts, and soybeans are good sources of vitamin B6.

Vitamin B12 (Cianocobalamine)

Vitamin B12 is the only one containing **cobalt.** It is only produced by microorganisms as bacteria, from which it passes to animals. These store the vitamin B12 in the liv-

71

Avocados are very rich in iron and proteins, aside from having a good percentage of fats.

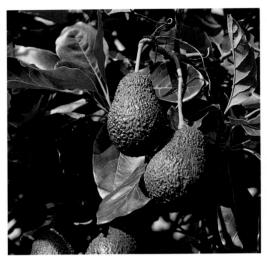

er. Plants do not produce B_{12}, but may contain it if they become contaminated with B_{12}-synthesizing bacteria.

Function

Together with folic acid it is indispensable for the formation of **blood cells,** especially the erythrocytes, as well as for the proper operation of the **nervous system.** Its *lack* results in an especially serious type of **anemia,** called **pernicious,** as well as the degeneration of the nervous fibers in the spinal cord.

Vitamin B₁₂ and the Vegetarian Diet

Up to a few years ago, the only known source of vitamin B_{12} was the liver of mammals, followed by meat, fish, eggs and dairy products. The lack of vitamin B_{12} in vegetables has been one of the most serious objections that have been raised against the strict vegetarian diet.

Today we know that, by bacterial contamination, the spirula algae contains an abundance of vitamin B_{12}, and in smaller quantities brewer's yeast and beer. Small quantities of B_{12} are also found in *tempeh* and other soy products. Some researchers states that most of the B_{12} contained in spirula, algae, and other vegetal food is an inactive form of the true vitamin B_{12}.

Nevertheless, even in the case of **strict vegetarians,** research has demonstrated that nutritional B_{12} deficiencies resulting from insufficient intake are very rare. The poor Asian diet, totally vegetable, provides 0.5 micrograms per day, which according to some authors, is sufficient. Millions of Hindus follow it[1] without suffering from pernicious anemia or showing any other manifestations of lack of vitamin B_{12}.

The average US diet supplies 5-15 daily µg of vitamin B_{12}, much more than the minimum requirements estimated as between 0.3 to 0.65 µg.[2] A dietary intake of 1 µg daily can be expected to sustain normal people but for extra security the Recommended Daily Allowance has been established in 2 µg.[3]

From where do strict vegetarians obtain vitamin B₁₂, since it is so scarce in the larger part of the plant

1. JATHAR, V.S. Vitamin B₁₂ and vegetarianism in India. *Acta Haematologica,* **53:** 90-97 (1975).
2. HERBERT, V. Recommended dietary intakes of vitamin B₁₂ in humans. *American Journal of Clinical Nutrition,* **45:** 671-678 (1987).
3. BAKER, S.J. Evidence regarding the minimal daily requirement of dietary vitamin B₁₂. *American Journal of Clinical Nutrition,* **34:** 2423-2433 (1981).

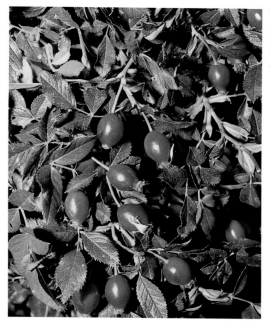

The wild rose (dog rose) grows spontaneously in mountains and valleys, and is one of the richest foods in vitamin C (600 mg per each 100 grams). This fruit is ingested in the form of jam or drinks.

taminate certain foods such as algae, yeasts, wheat germ and possibly others.[4] The less hygiene practiced on food handling (which often happens in impoverished countries), the greater the probability that it will be contaminated by bacteria which produce vitamin B_{12}. Therefore, fortunately, the lack of this vitamin is not as frequent as some would have you believe.

In a lactovegetarian or ovolactovegetarian diet there is no risk of vitamin B_{12} deficiency. Nevertheless, those following a strict vegetarian diet should not become careless in the acquisition of vitamin B_{12}, for the two sources which we just mentioned are not controllable, and at least theoretically there is the risk of a deficit if the intestinal absorption is not correct. In these cases, it may be necessary to take a nutritional supplement.

Vegetarians who use milk or eggs, even though it may not be on a daily basis, also have no problems relating to the lack of this vitamin, for the needs of vitamin B_{12} are sufficiently covered by these products of animal origin. It should be said that the **ovolactovegetarian diet** is recognized *without reservation* by all researchers in nutrition as **healthful** and **complete** (see page 116).

foods? Recent research confirms two ways:

- From **bacteria** found in the **large intestine** (colon), which synthesizes vitamin B_{12} in great quantities. Though it's true that the capacity for absorption in the large intestine is quite limited, it would seem that it is sufficient to allow the passage of a certain quantity of vitamin B_{12} to the blood. We know that **vitamin B_{12}** is not the only one produced by intestinal bacteria: **vitamin K** is another example. It could be possible that bacteria usually colonizing the mouth would be able to produce sufficient B_{12} to satisfy daily needs.

- From **the microorganisms** which **produce vitamin B_{12}** which habitually con-

4. PASSMORE AND EASTWOOD. *Human Nutrition and Dietetics*, 1986.

Vitamin C
in some foods

Food	Content in miligrams per 100 grams	Quantity of food in g providing the recommended daily allowance (60 mg)
Wild Rose	600	10
Kiwi	98	61
Peppers	89	67
Raspberries	25	240
Oranges	53.2	113
Lemons	53	113
Fresh peas	40	150
Cabbage	32	188
Spinach	28	214
Mangoes	27.7	217
Tomatoes	23.4	256
Radishes	22.8	263
Pineapple	15	400
Alfalfa	8	750
Cherries	7	857
Onions	6	1,000
Cereals	0	-
Milk	0.94	6,383
Salmon	0	-
meat	0	-
Eggs	0	-

Vitamin C
(Ascorbic Acid)

For centuries **scurvy** was one of the most frequent debilitating diseases, especially during the winter months in which, on trips on the high seas, the diet was monotonously based on cereals and dried meat or sausages. In 1928, **Szent Györgyi,** a Hungarian chemist, discovered vitamin C, and it was proven that it abounds in vegetables and fruits.

Vitamin C is the **vegetarian vitamin** par excellence. No one whose nourishment is based on vegetables will lack vitamin C. Eating only one orange which contains about 90 milligrams of vitamin C, or a tomato, which may have as much as 130 milligrams, will cover the daily allowance of 60 mg recommended by the US National Research Council. Meat, fish and eggs are very poor in or totally lack ascorbic acid. Milk has a small amount, enough for a baby, but not enough for a child or an adult.

Vitamin C
daily needs

Children . . . . 40 - 45 mg

Male adults. . . . . 60 mg

Female adults . . . . 60 mg

Pregnant. . . . . 70 mg

Lactating . . . . 95 mg

In the case of infection, wounds, or surgery, the daily requirement increases considerably, and it is well to increase daily allowance by the use of fruit juices, vegetables or nutritional supplements.

Vitamin C is very sensitive to heat and light, so when foods are cooked or fried, they lose a good part of their content. The same happens to canned products. This is another reason for daily use of fresh and raw foods such as fruits and salads.

Functions

Vitamin C activates the functions of all the cells. It is a *powerful* **antioxidant,** and some suggest that it *impedes* the biochemical processes of cellular **aging** (and possibly, also, cancer), which are mostly of an oxidative type. It *favors* the **absorption** of **iron** in the intestines, contributes to the formation of **defenses** against infections, neutralizes blood toxins, intervenes in the healing of wounds, and performs many other physiologically important functions.

Its lack gives way to a disease called **scurvy,** which is identified by weakness, a tendency toward infections, anemia, and hemorrhages in the gums and the skin.

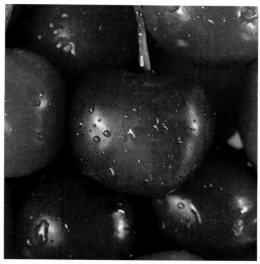

Cherries contain a balanced portion of vitamin C and iron, which favors the absorption of this mineral.

Vitamin D
daily needs

Children and young	10 µg (400 UI)
Male adults	5 µg (200 UI)
Female adults	5 µg (200 UI)
Pregnant	10 µg (400 UI)
Lactating	10 µg (400 UI)

Sunbathing in the sun (naked) for one minute per day, or walking one hour in the open air (dressed) is sufficient for the skin to synthesize the required daily allowance of vitamin D.
Only in regions where the sun does not shine for long periods of time, especially in the winter, are supplements of vitamin D indicated.

At the present time scurvy is very rare. *At times* it will occur when there is a **partial lack** of vitamin C brought on by a lack of fresh fruits and and raw vegetables in the diet. These are manifested by minor symptoms which may not be perceived: abnormal tiredness, both physical and mental, easy bleeding, propensity toward infections, and slow growth in children, among others.

Vitamin D (Calciferol)

The anti-rickets power of cod fish oil was already known at the end of the eighteenth century. The liposoluble substance responsible for this effect was isolated in 1920, and it was called vitamin D.

Vitamin D presents itself in two distinct chemical forms:

Vitamins that Are Not Stored

Vitamin C does not accumulate within the body, and therefore must be ingested daily. Fat-soluble vitamins such as A and D accumulate in the liver, so it is possible to pass several weeks, and even months, without sun bathing to activate them.

But this does not occur with **vitamin C** and other **water-solubles**, because they are not stored in the body and **must be ingested daily.** For this reason it is important to eat fresh fruit and vegetables every day.

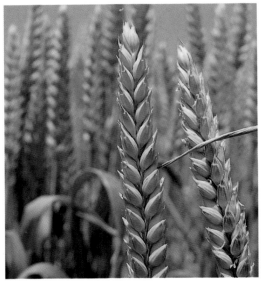

Wheat germ, as is the case with other cereals and seeds, is the most important source of vitamin E.

- **Vitamin D₃ (cholecalciferol)**, which is formed naturally in man and animals, especially in fish, and is stored in the **liver.** Under the influence of the rays of the sun it is synthesized in the basal skin layer, beginning with a derivative of cholesterol (7-dehydrocholesterol).
- **Vitamin D₂ (ergocalciferol)**, which is produced artificially in the laboratory and is used to enrich foods in vitamin D, and in pharmaceutical preparations.

The major part of vitamin D which circulates throughout the blood is synthesized in our own skin. In fact, if we are exposed to the **sun,** even in small quantities, there is no need to depend on food for this vitamin.[5]

Functions

Vitamin D *facilitates* the ***absorption*** of **calcium** in the intestine, as well as its storage in the bones. When there is insufficient vitamin D in the body, bones become soft, becoming deformed because they cannot support the weight of the body. This disease is known as rickets.

Foods that Contain Vitamin D

Fish liver (cod) is the external source most abundant in vitamin D. Also fish meat, milk, butter and eggs have it in small quantities. Some researchers underline the fact that vegetable products such as avocados, bananas, cocoa or wheat germ also contain it although this does not seem to be generally accepted.

At any rate, according to the recommendations of the WHO/FAO, the ingestion is only necessary when there is no access to

---

5. FAO / OMS, Studies on Nutrition No. 28. *Manual on the Nutritional Needs of Man.* Rome, Food and Agriculture Organization, 1975, pages 35, 36.

Vitamin E
in some foods

Food	Content in miligrams per 100 grams	Quantity of food in g providing the recommended daily allowance (10 mg)
Corn oil	192	10
Sunflower oil	51	39
Almonds	24	83
Wheat germ	14	143
Olive oil	12	167
Nuts	2.6	769
Avocados	2.3	870
Soybeans	1.95	1,026
Spinach	1.89	1,058
Peaches	0.7	2,857
Peppers	0.69	2,899
Raspberries	0.45	4,444
Butter	1.58	1,266
Eggs	1.05	1,905
Grouper (fish)	0.5	4,000
Liver	0.34	5,882
Chicken breast	0.3	6,667
Lean pork meat	0.29	6,897
Leg of lamb	0.21	9,524
Milk	0.1	20,000

the sun, especially children who live in cold climates. So with the small quantities that may be contained in the foods, and a *bit* of **sunshine** each day, all our vitamin D needs are covered except in disease conditions.

Danger of Overdosing

During the 1950 and 60's the fad of enriching certain foods with **vitamin D** aimed at little children became prevalent. This brought on many cases of *overdosing,* with the resulting calcification of the kidneys and heart which led to several deaths.[6]

A dose four times the daily requirement is toxic. We are dealing with a "dangerous" vitamin, and it is perhaps for this reason nature has it in such small quantities. The body produces the dosage that it really needs with a little exposure to the sun each day, and so there is no risk of overdosage.

Vitamin E (Tocopherol)

It is a fat-soluble vitamin the same as A, D and K, but different from the first two. It is much more abundant in plant foods, than in those of animal origin, and presents less risk of toxicity in high dosages than other fat-soluble vitamins.

6. FAO / OMS, Studies on Nutrition No. 28. *Manual on the Nutritional Needs of Man.* Rome, Food and Agriculture Organization, 1975, page 35.

Vitamin E
daily needs

Children	6 - 7 mg
Male adults.	10 mg
Female adults.	8 mg
Pregnant	10 mg
Lactating	12 mg

Functions

Vitamin E plays an important part in the metabolism. Its most outstanding activities are:

- Protects the cells **against** aging, possibly because of its **antioxidant** action.

- Exerts **protective** action against **cancer.** Laboratory animals to which abundant vitamin E has been given, are more resistant to the action of cancerous agents than those who take none.

- Takes part in the formation of reproductive cells (spermatozoids and ovules). It **improves** the fertility of the **semen.** It is recommended to women who have a tendency to **abort.**

- Facilitates the good operation of the **nervous system** and of the **pituitary gland,** which controls the hormone production of the body.

Sources

Vitamin E abounds throughout nature, especially in **plant foods.** Cereal germs, vegetable oils, and nuts are the best sources of vitamin E. Meat has but little vitamin E. As can be seen, the vegetarian diet, especially if whole cereals are eaten (vitamin E is in the germ) provides large doses of this interesting vitamin, which fulfills so many functions within our body.

It should be made clear that not all flours which are called "whole" because they have a darker color, contain the cereal germ. In some cases the so-called whole flour is no more than a mixture of white flour and bran. The authentic whole flours, which include the germ, tend to become rancid very soon, which makes it necessary to use them freshly milled. Cereal flakes tend to include the germ. It is well to keep these details in mind to evaluate the quality of the cereals and their flours.

Vitamin K

It is a fat-soluble vitamin which acts in the liver leading to the synthesis of the proteins needed for the coagulation of blood. It acts in the prevention of **hemorrhaging.** Its absence is manifested in certain diseases of the digestive system, or in the case of premature births.

Sources

Vitamin K comes from two sources:

- **Intestinal bacteria,** which produce it in sufficient quantity for the daily needs. High or prolonged doses of antibiotics may destroy some of these "friendly" bac-

Vitamin K
in some foods

Food	Content in micrograms (µg) per 100 grams	Quantity of food in g providing the recommended daily allowance (80 µg)
Spinach	558	14.3
Broccoli	325	24.6
Turnip greens	296	27
Lettuce	290	27.6
Cabbage	246	32.5
Peas	244	32.8
Ox liver	292	27.4
Cheese	187	42.8
Milk	152	52.6

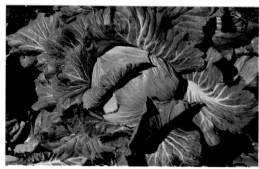

Cabbage is a good source of vitamin K and folic acid.

teria which are normally found in the intestines, and can provoke a lack of vitamins.

- **Foods,** especially vegetables like turnips and cabbage.

Other Vitamins*

Up to twenty other substances are known aside from those mentioned above, indispensable in small doses for the human body, and which the body is not capable of synthesizing. All are found in the vegetable kingdom, and in smaller proportion in milk, eggs, and meat.

Niacin: It plays an essential role to play in chemical mechanisms through which the cells *take advantage* of the **energy** proceeding from the **nutrients** (carbohydrates, fats and proteins). It is found in brewer's yeast, whole cereals, fruit, vegetables, peanuts and legumes, especially soybeans.

Its lack produces a disease known as **pellagra,** still quite frequent in areas of the world in which poverty has obliged people to follow poor diets, for example, diets based on corn. Pellagra is the disease of the **three D's:** **d**iarrhea, **d**ermatitis (inflammation of the skin) and **d**ementia.

Folic acid and folates: They act together with vitamin B$_{12}$, favoring the production of **erythrocytes** (red corpuscles) in the bone marrow. Its importance during the time of **pregnancy** has recently been proven, since its lack, especially during the first months, provokes malformation in the fetus.

The daily needs are 200 micrograms for children and adults, and 400 for pregnant women.

It is amply found among vegetables (folate comes from the latin word *folium,* leaf) so that a vegetarian diet guarantees the daily needs. Foods that are the richest in folic acid and folates are: spinach, asparagus, lettuce, endives, avocados, bananas, oranges and nuts.

Nevertheless there are three situations which increase the need for folic acid and folates, making it necessary to give special attention to consuming enough **vegetables,** *especially **raw*** ones:

- During **pregnancy,**
- When using **alcoholic beverages** (alcohol resists the action of folic acid)
- When certain **medicines** are taken, especially the barbiturates against epilepsy, and anticancer chemotherapy.

---

* Although they are not considered to be true vitamins, the phytochemical substances which are found in vegetables also have preventive and even curative functions. (See next page).

Phytochemical Elements

When, around a decade ago, the specialists in nutrition thought they had identified all the components in food, a new group of natural ingredients in fruit, cereals and vegetables started being discovered. They are substances that have a **preventive** and even **healing action,** explaining the medicinal properties of vegetable foods. They are true **natural medicines** that vegetables possess, which modern chemical analysis methods are allowing to be identified in a growing number.

Phytochemical elements are also simply called phytochemicals, accompanying substances, non-nutritional substances, medicofoods (contraction of medicines and foods), metanutrients (because they go beyond classical nutrients: carbohydrates, proteins, fats, minerals and vitamins).

Characteristics:

- They are found **exclusively in vegetables,** particularly in fruit, vegetables and cereals.

- They are found in **very small** amounts.

- They **do not** provide **calories.**

- Many of them are **natural pigments** that color the vegetables.

- They are **antioxidants;** that is to say, **they protect** the organism **against free radicals,** aggressive chemical molecules causing cellular ageing, degenerative diseases and cancer.

Types:

These are some of the phytochemical elements that have been identified:

- **Flavonoids:** They protect the **arteries** and the **heart.** They are particularly found in citric fruits, apples, onions and in grapes.

- **Antocyanines:** They protect the **heart,** they tone the venous **circulation,** and they regenerate the **retina.** Black grapes, blackberries, pomegranates and bilberries are the best sources of these.

- **Isoflavons:** They prevent osteoporosis and they protect against **cancer** (particularly breast and prostate cancer). They are found in soya and in some of its derivatives such as soya drink or milk and tofu (soya cheese).

- **Sulphurous compounds:** They are the parts that form the hot, spicy essence of cabbages and radishes. They are effective **anti-cancerigenic** elements.

- **Carotenoids:** They are orange-colored pigments that protect against **cancer,** as well as transforming into vitamin A. Carrots, oranges, tomatoes and mangoes are some of the best natural sources.

8

Minerals

AROUND TWENTY minerals are known that form a part of our bodies. Minerals make up 5% of the weight of our bodies, that is, about 3.5 kilos for a 70-kilo (154 lb) adult. Minerals are constantly being renovated within our bodies. Around 30 grams of minerals are eliminated each day through urine, feces, perspiration, and other secretions, and these must necessarily be replaced through food.

The most important source of minerals are the plant foods in their natural state, especially those originating in organic farming. Therefore, **flesh diets** and those based on **refined products** tend to be *deficient* in minerals. This is aggravated by the fact that the land becomes impoverished in minerals because of the intensive use of inorganic fertilizers. Actually, it is quite possible that the products that we purchase in the food stores contain less minerals than they should have according to the composition of food charts.

If it runs, don't eat it.

ENGLISH PROVERB

Calcium
in some foods

Food	Content in miligrams per 100 grams	Quantity of food in g providing the recommended daily allowance (800 mg)	Food	Content in miligrams per 100 grams	Quantity of food in g providing the recommended daily allowance (800 mg)
Sesame seeds	975	82	Cured cheese (average)	1,011	79
Soybeans	277	289	Natural yogurt	121	661
Almonds	266	301	Milk	119	672
Hazel nuts	188	426	Cottage cheese	68.5	1,168
Spinach	99	808	Fresh cheese	68.5	1,168
Nuts	94	851	Liquid cream	64.6	1,238
Oat flakes	54	1,481	Eggs	49	1,633
Endive	52	1,538	Mother's milk	32	2,500
Peanut butter	41	1,951	Cod fish	16	5,000
Whole wheat flour	34	2,353	Pork	15	5,333
			Veal	15	5,333
White wheat flour	15	5,333	Salmon	12	6,667
Rice	9	8,889	Chicken	12	6,667
Soy milk	4	20,000	Lamb	10	8,000

Therefore we should pay close attention to the minerals in our diet, *especially* **calcium** and **iron.**

Calcium

It is the most abundant mineral in the body, whose salts form the substance that hardens the skeleton and teeth. The body of an adult contains between 1 and 1.5 kilos of calcium, the larger part of which (99%) is found in bones and teeth, and a

Calcium
daily needs

Children . . . . 800 mg

Youth 11-24. . . . . 1,200 mg

Males adults . . . . 800 mg

Females adults . . . . 800 mg

Pregnant . . . . 1,200 mg

Lactating . . . . 1,200 mg

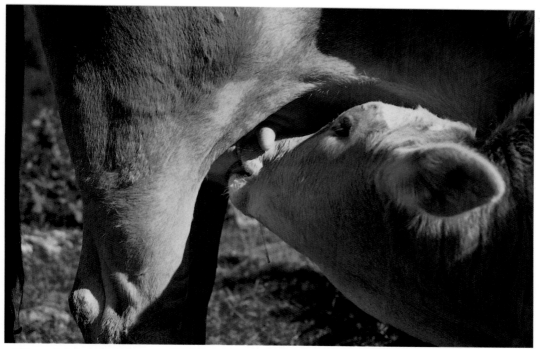

Milk and dairy products are the best source of calcium among the animal products. But cow milk has a large amount of fat, needed for the development of the calf, but not for human beings, especially adults. Sesame seeds and nuts (almonds, hazelnuts) provide as much or more calcium than milk, with the added advantage that they contain no saturated fat nor cholesterol.

small part (1%) in the blood and the rest of the organism.

In addition to being a part of the skeleton, calcium performs other interesting functions in the body:

- It intervenes in the transmission of **nerve impulses,** especially in the **heart,** thus maintaining the cardiac rhythm.

- It is needed to maintain a normal **coagulation** of the **blood.**

- It regulates the **basic-acid balance** of blood, keeping it from becoming too acid. In this way it neutralizes the acid which normally is produced through the metabolism of proteins.

Calcium needs **vitamin D** to be absorbed into the intestines and thus be passed on to the blood.

The deficiency of calcium is first manifested in a condition known as tetany, which is characterized by muscular cramps which can actually become spasms. When this persists, it causes changes in the heart rhythm (palpitations), nervous irritability, loss of the normal hardness of the bones (rickets in children, and osteoporosis or osteomalacia in adults), pain in the joints and loss of teeth.

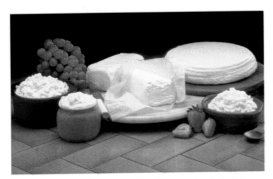

Cottage cheese and milk curd contain abundant proteins and have very little fat. Their proportion of calcium is as high as 300 mg per 100 grams.

Calcium in the Vegetarian Diet

Calcium is found in **plant foods,** especially in nuts and legumes. A diet based on fruit, cereals, and vegetables provides more than enough calcium needed by the body, with notable advantages over the meat diet. Among animal foods, only milk and its derivatives have important amounts of calcium, but it is very rare in meat and fish.

It is well to remember that **oxalic acid** contained in some foods may slow down the absorption of calcium, as this combination forms insoluble salts (calcium oxalate). Though food rich in oxalic acid, such as cacao, spinach and celery, also have abundant calcium, it is well to take them in small quantities when a diet high in calcium is required.

Phosphorus

Practically all of the phosphorus in the body is found in the bones and teeth, combined with **calcium.**

The quantity of phosphorus that is in the diet must be related to calcium. Phosphorus is found widely distributed among all foods, both vegetable and animal, so there is no risk of insufficiency.

To the contrary, the *main **problem*** with phosphorus is its **excess** in relation to the amount of calcium. This happens especially in diets overloaded with meat, for meat contains a great deal of phosphorus and very little calcium (up to ten times more in pork). This excess of phosphorus in the meat diet causes calcium to be less utilized, and is another factor which may explain the *frequency* of **osteoporosis** among women who eat *large amounts* of **meat.**

Plant foods as well as milk and eggs maintain the quantity of phosphorus in a much more balanced relationship with calcium. Thus in an ovolactovegetarian diet there is less danger of taking in too much phosphorus.

Iron

The organism of an adult contains between three and four grams of iron. This, of course, is a very small quantity, but it performs function a of vital importance. The larger part of iron is found in the blood, forming part of the **hemoglobin,** which

continues on page 86

Almonds are among the richest foods in calcium (266 mg per 100 g). Their content in phosphorus (454 mg per 100 g) maintains a balanced proportion with calcium.

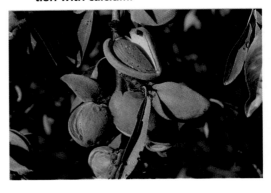

An excess of protein leads to a loss of calcium

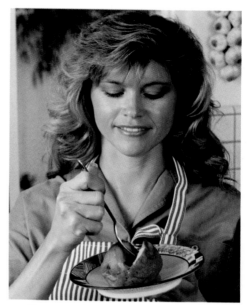

The use of meat and cured cheeses favors osteoporosis. On the other hand, a balanced vegetarian diet protects from this disease.

It's important to emphasize a fact in relation to calcium. **Proteins** are **necessary** so that calcium will remain fixed in the bones, but an **excess** has a **harmful** effect. A report by a group of experts of the WHO*, emphasizes that in **a diet rich in proteins or in common salt the loss of calcium increases,** so that the body is impoverished in this mineral. This seems to be an important factor in the cause of **osteoporosis,** a disease that affects millions of women in developed countries.

This curious phenomenon can be explained as follows: The more proteins ingested, especially if they are of animal origin (in particular meat and cured cheese), the more **blood is acidified** by the action of lactic and uric acids which are formed when proteins are metabolized. This forces the body to use part of its calcium reserves to compensate for the excess of acid. For, as we already have said, one of the functions of calcium is to maintain the balance between the acid and alkaline substances in the blood.

Furthermore, calcium forms soaps which cannot be absorbed by the intestines as it binds with the fatty acids coming from the digestion of fats. **Therefore a rich supply of fats makes the absorption of calcium difficult.**

It must be understood, however, that aside from this, osteoporosis has other causes of a hormonal or metabolic nature. But it has been demonstrated that the use of meat in large quantities and cured cheese (because of their richness in proteins and fats) increases the loss of calcium, and worsens the illness. On the other hand, a **balanced vegetarian diet** which contains the needed proteins has an **alkalizing** effect (as opposed to meat), diminishes the loss of calcium and acts as a **preventive** of **osteoporosis,** especially if it is accompanied with **physical exercise.**

---

* WHO, Technical Report Series, No. 797, *(Diet, Nutrition, and the Prevention of Chronic Diseases). Report of a WHO Study Group.* Geneva, World Health Organization, 1990, page 82.

Iron
in some foods

Food	Content in miligrams per 100 grams	Quantity of food in g providing the recommend-ed daily allowance (10 mg)	Food	Content in miligrams per 100 grams	Quantity of food in g providing the recommend-ed daily allowance (10 mg)
Dried spirula (algae)	28.5	35	Asparagus	0.87	1,149
Brewer's yeast	18	56	Potatoes	0.76	1,316
Soybean	16	63	Cabbage	0.59	1,695
Sesame seed	15	67	Apricots	0.54	1,852
White beans	10	100	Carrots	0.5	2,000
Lentils	9.02	111	Figs	0.37	2,703
Pollen	9	111	Grapes	0.26	3,846
Pistachios	6.8	147	Apples	0.18	5,556
Sunflower seeds	6.77	148	Peaches	0.11	9,091
Chickpeas	6.2	161	Prunes	0.1	10,000
Oats	4.7	213	Liver	4.8	208
Almonds	3.7	270	Beef	1.8	556
Wheat	3.2	313	Lamb	1.77	565
Pine nuts	3.1	323	Eggs	1.4	714
Spinach	2.7	370	Chicken	0.89	1,124
Nuts	2.4	417	Pork	0.89	1,124
Leeks	2.1	476	Tuna in oil	0.65	1,538
Peas	1.5	667	Semi-fat cheese	0.33	3,030
Mushrooms	1.2	833			
Green beans	1.04	962	Milk	0.05	20,000
Avocado	1.02	980	Yogurt	0.05	20,000

Vitamin C, abundant in foods coming from the vegetable kingdom, facilitates the absorption of iron into the intestines. This is one reason why foods based on plants amply satisfy the daily needs for iron.

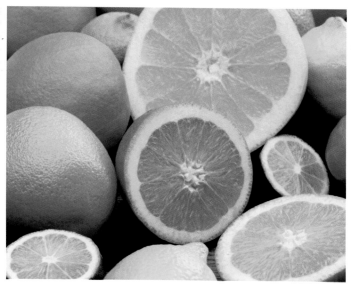

continues from page 84

causes the typical red color and allows the transportation of **oxygen** from the lungs to all the cells.

Iron does not exist as an isolated chemical element within the body, which would behave as an authentic poison, but combines with proteins, especially the one called **ferritin.**

Iron daily needs	
Children.	10 mg
Males 11-18	12 mg
Male adults	10 mg
Females 11-50	15 mg
Females 51+	10 mg
Pregnant	30 mg
Lactating	15 mg

Daily Need of Iron

The major part of iron found in the body recycles itself, so that under normal conditions the loss of this mineral is minimal. Iron is lost when cells scale off the skin and the mucosa linings covering the inside of the digestive and urinary systems. This loss is about 1.0 milligram per day for an adult.

In certain situations the need for iron increases:

- **Menstruating women** lose an average of two more milligrams of iron per day with menstrual blood, which means that during the period women lose three times more iron than normally.

- **During pregnancy** and **breast feeding** the need for iron increases, but is compensated by the fact that there is no menstrual loss. So the need for iron is the same for a woman during the menstrual period as when she is pregnant or is breast feeding.

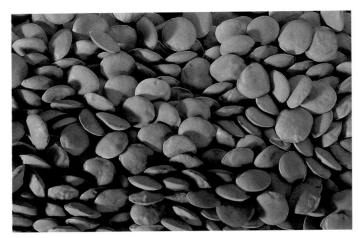

Lentils are very rich in protein and iron, to the point that they exceed meat in both nutrients. Its proteins supplement well those found in cereals, for example, rice.

- During **adolescence** the need for iron increases because of growth and the beginning of menstruation in young women.

- Any abnormal **hemorrhage** causes a significant loss of iron which may easily produce anemia.

Iron in **plants** is found in the form of **ferric salts,** while those in **animals,** also called *heme*-**iron,** appears in the form of **ferrous salts.** Both types of iron are absorbed with difficulty in the intestines, to the point that only 10% to 20% of the iron coming from the plant is absorbed, and 30% of the iron found in meat or animal foods. Because of this, when calculating daily needs, thought should be given to ingesting ten times more iron than we really need as a measure of security.

Iron in the Vegetarian Diet

Iron is found widely throughout all animal and vegetable foods, and a varied diet abundantly provides for the daily needs, including that of women.

The lesser absorption of iron coming from plants is compensated in two ways:

- The ***concentration*** of iron found in **plant foods** is *higher* than in **meats,** except liver. Milk hardly has any iron.

- It has been demonstrated that **vitamin C,** very abundant in the vegetarian diet, greatly *increases* the ***absorption*** of **iron,** even doubling it. This is an important reason for including vegetables and/or fruit, rich in vitamin C, in each meal.

Against popular belief, there is no reason for vegetarian diets to be poor in iron. The fact is that anemia caused by poor nutrition is quite frequent, affecting both those who eat meat and those who are vegetarians. For a time it was thought that meat was necessary because of its iron content, and those who did not eat meat ran the risk of having anemia. But today we know that the **vegetarian diet** is ***superior*** in its **iron** content and that its absorption presents no problems if fresh foods rich in **vitamin C** are consumed.

Nuts, legumes and cereals contain more iron than meat, except liver. Soybean flour from which vegetarian meat is made, has three times more iron than beef (the meat with the highest iron content). The WHO

Custard apples are a very tasty subtropical fruit which contain important quantities of calcium (15 mg per 100 grams) and iron (0.6 mg per 100 grams).

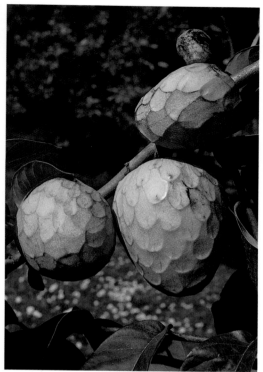

recommends the abundant use of peaches, apricots, prunes, grapes, and raisins as excellent sources of iron for their easy digestion and absorption.[1] Spirula algae, brewer's yeast, sesame seed, and pollen are, together with soybeans, the vegetarian foods richest in iron.

Persons who have low iron absorption, or when the daily requirements increase, could well use a supplement of this mineral. Aside from pharmaceutical preparations, there are also those coming from plant extracts.

Iodine

The body needs iodine to synthesize the hormones produced in the thyroid gland. These hormones fulfill important metabolic functions:

- *Accelerate* the **combustion** of **nutrients** that provide energy (carbohydrates, fats and proteins).

- Are indispensable for the development of the **nervous system** in **children,** so that when there is a scarcity of iodine, a form of mental retardation (cretinism) may develop.

When an adult suffers from a lack of iodine, the thyroid hypertrophies itself (increases in size) in order to compensate for a lack in the production of sufficient thyroid hormones. This increase is called simple goiter (there are other causes of goiter).

The needs for iodine are very small: 0.14 milligrams per day. Normally fruit and vegetables supply sufficient iodine if the soil where they have grown contains it. But there are lands deficient in iodine (generally those far removed from the coast) and others which have become impoverished in this mineral because of intensive farming, which depletes the mineral reserves in the soil. Because of this, deficiencies are not rare. To avoid them it is important to:

- Use **sea salt** or salt which has been enriched with iodine.

- Eat food **algae.**

1. FAO / WHO, Studies on Nutrition, No. 28. *Manual on the Nutricional Needs of Man.* Rome, Food and Agriculture Organization, 1975, page 62.

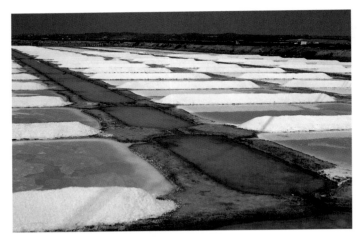

Marine salt provides, aside from sodium chloride, other mineral salts of iodine and magnesium. Because of this, its use is preferable to mined or refined salt, although their use with food should not pass six grams per day, according to the recommendations of the WHO. Those who suffer hypertension and who have heart problems should not use more than three grams per day.

Fish also have an abundance of iodine, although their use is not indispensable in satisfying the daily needs.

Magnesium

The body of an adult contains between 20 and 25 grams of magnesium. It is part of the bone structure together with calcium and phosphorus, although in a much smaller proportion. Magnesium is an essential component of the main pigment in the vegetable kingdom, **chlorophyll,** the same as iron is to the blood hemoglobin.

Magnesium has increased in importance during recent years, due to the fact that many physiological functions have been discovered in which it plays a decisive role.

It frequently happens that ordinary diet provides insufficient quantities of this important mineral. This is due to the infrequent use of whole cereals and nuts, which are rich in magnesium, as well as the impoverishment of this mineral in the soil. The perma-

nent abuse of nitrogenated fertilizer in intensive farming cause biochemical imbalance in the soil and as a result, in the plants that grow in them. Plants do not have the quantity of minerals which they should have, especially magnesium, which is one of the most sensitive to soil impoverishment.

For this reason special attention should be given to magnesium and, in certain cases of deficiency, resort to the use of supplementary minerals such as chloride of magnesium.

It should be remembered that the recommended daily allowance of magnesium established by the US National Research Council, are 350 mg for male adults and 280 mg for female adults. Although the use of large doses of magnesium salts does not have harmful effects, it has not been proven that it has any special therapeutic action. The excess of magnesium is eliminated with the feces, having a laxative effect.

The use of **magnesium supplements** in the form of salts is indicated in the following cases:

Magnesium
in some foods

Food	Content in miligrams per 100 grams	Quantity of food in g providing the recommended daily allowance (350 mg)
Sunflower seeds	354	99
Almonds	296	118
Soybeans	280	125
Walnuts	169	207
Whole wheat flour	138	254
Spinach	79	443
Chocolate	65	538
Lima beans	58	603
Bananas	29	1,207
White wheat flour	22	1,591
Potatoes	21	1,667
Figs	17	2,059
Papaya	10	3,500
Oranges	10	3,500
Cod	32	1,094
Grouper	31	1,129
Leg of lamb	23	1,522
Ham	18	1,944
Milk	13	2,692
Eggs	10	3,500

Magnesium
daily needs

Children.	80 - 170 mg
Males 15-18.	400 mg
Male adults	350 mg
Females 15-18.	300 mg
Females adults.	280 mg
Pregnant	320 mg
Lactating	355 mg

- When there is a risk that the **food supply** is **insufficient,** because refined food make up a large portion of the diet.
- In times of life when there is an increase in daily needs (**growth, pregnancy, breast feeding**).
- When the **intestinal absorption** is **altered** by different digestive problems, for example, colitis or bowel surgery.

Functions

It acts as a catalyst of many chemical reactions which take place in the organism, related to the combustion of nutrients and the production of energy. It exerts an especially important function in the **nervous system,** regulating the transmission of its impulses to the peripheral nerves.

The lack of magnesium reveals itself in different ways:

- A general sense of fatigue.
- Muscular cramps, rigidity, spasms in the eyelids or in other muscles (a phenomenon known as muscular fasciculation).
- Neurological alterations with a tendency toward spasms in different organs which are manifested by: stomach aches, irritat-

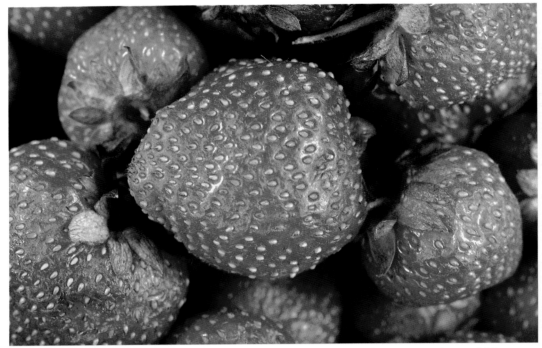

Strawberries contain a wide range of mineral salts, among them magnesium, which makes them a diuretic valuable in the treatment of kidney diseases.

ed colon, menstrual cramps (dysmenorrhoea), a feeling of tightness in the chest, and heart palpitations among others.

Nuts, cereals, legumes and vegetables are the most important sources of magnesium. A varied vegetarian diet can more than satisfy the need for magnesium, especially if it comes from biological cultivation where organic fertilizers which contain a wide variety of minerals are used.

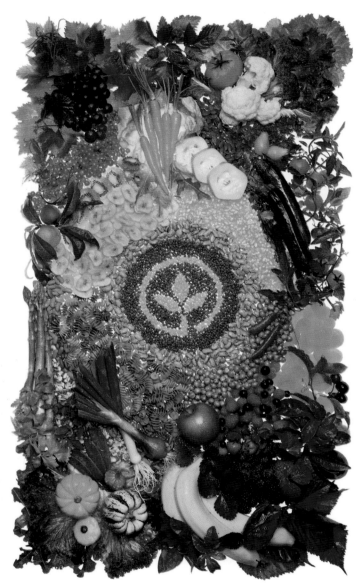

In diets which include a variety of vegetables of a suitable quality and quantity there is no need for vitamin and mineral supplements. This type of supplement is only necessary in the case of illness or when there are obvious deficiencies. A diet based on vegetables more than satisfies all mineral and trace element requirements.

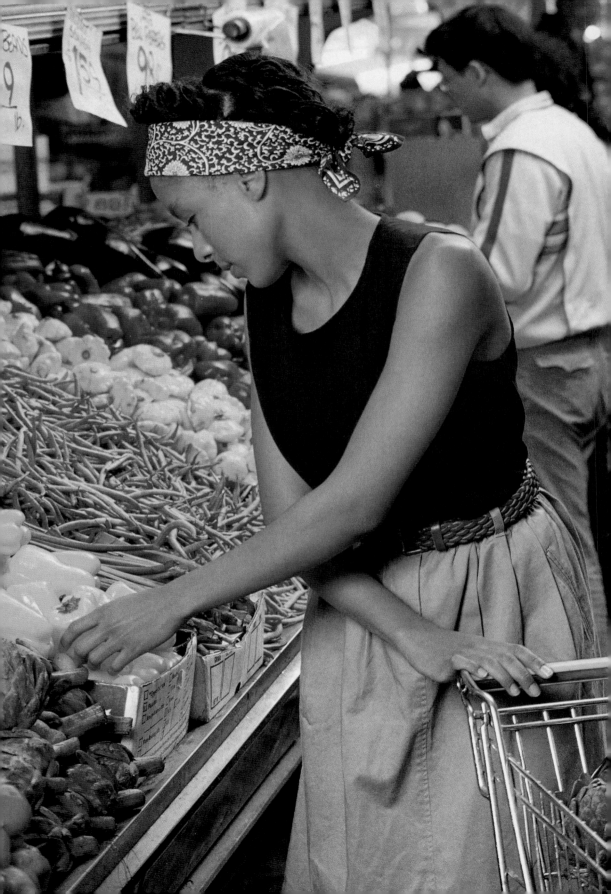

9

A Novelty With a Long Tradition

THE MEDIA bombards us daily with messages on what we should eat. But it often happens that what they recommend is not the most healthful. Therefore, what should we eat in order to maintain health?

The European Code Against Cancer, developed by a committee of experts from all countries of the European Community, recommends in Point 3 (point 5 in the first version of the Code): *"Eat frequently: fruit, fresh vegetables and cereals with a high fiber content."*

In order to maintain good health, we should mostly eat foods of plant origin. Fruit, grains, and vegetables (including greens, legumes and tubers), constitute the basic diet of the human family. With them it is possible not only to be well nourished, but further, to prevent many diseases such as cancer.

To maintain health, fruit and fresh vegetables must be the fundamental part of our food.

MAHATMA GANDHI
Liberator of India
1869-1948

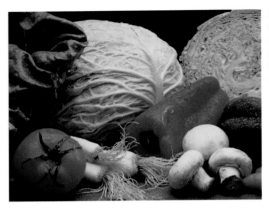

Fruit, cereals, and vegetables constituted the basic diet of many peoples, underlining the fact that the first human beings were vegetarian.

The Original Diet

A diet rich in fruits, cereals, and vegetables, now recommended by the European Community as ideal to prevent cancer and other degenerative diseases, was precisely the original diet of mankind. The book of Genesis, one of the world's literary gems, written by Moses around 3,500 years ago, says in its first chapter, verse 29: *"Behold, I have given you every herb bearing seed, which is upon the face of all the earth, and every tree, in the which is the fruit of a tree yielding seed; to you it shall be for meat."*

Surprising, isn't it? Man was not carnivorous, but a vegetarian at the beginning. It is possibly thanks to this that the human race has survived, for today we know that the vegetarian diet is healthier and recommended over a flesh diet.

In the oldest genealogical records which have been kept (the book of Genesis) a very important fact can be observed: When man abandoned the original vegetarian diet, and began to include flesh foods in his diet, the length of his life began to diminish ... until today!

There are many peoples who throughout history, for various reasons, have followed this original and basic diet for mankind. It is suitable to remember these and thus verify the beneficial effects upon health.

The Far East

Buddhism, Brahmanism and Hinduism, the great oriental religions, hold high the vegetarian diet. Nevertheless, the believers who do not follow it are not penalized. Buddhist monks eat foods of vegetable origin, which, furthermore, are those which are more easily available. Buddha taught that no creature should ever be killed. The first of the Buddhist Ten Precepts is *"avoid the destruction of life."* The principle of taking care of all living creatures without harming them, is a fundamental pillar of Hindu philosophy.

Several centuries before Christ, as Buddhism was losing its dominance in India, it was being introduced into China and came to be the religion of state in that great Empire. These are some of the outstanding popular proverbs of that time: *"Do not kill the ox that plows your field"*, *"Do not permit the voracity which gives way to the killing of animals."* Even today the principal products included in the Chinese diet are wheat, millet and corn in the north, while in the south the main food is rice. Meat and milk are used sporadically, when finances permit.

During the sixth and seventh centuries A.D. Buddhism was extended to Japan, where the basic diet was based on rice and beans. Only when circumstances permitted it, they consumed fish.

Nations in the Near East

Ancient Egyptians, known as *"bread eaters,"* cultivated cereals from the most ancient times. Studies which have been carried on, analyzing the intestinal contents of Egyptian mummies, reveal that their diet was basically of plant origin.

Although Persians were omnivorous, Porphyry (Greek philosopher and historian of the third century A.D.) tells how priests were not allowed to eat meat.

Around the year 1400 B.C. the ancient Israelites, various millenniums before scientific medicine, had by divine inspiration a rational group of norms referring to nutrition and hygiene, which are still valid today. Meat was tolerated as a reserve or exceptional food, and even then, with limitations. Pork was not considered to be fit for human consumption, neither shellfish, nor animal fats, nor blood, for example. Today we know that these foods are harmful to health because of their abundance of cholesterol, uric acid and animal toxins.

Middle East
The First Vegetarian Experiment in History

The Bible records in the book of Daniel a fact which has drawn the attention of students of nutrition: The Neo-Babylonian Empire conquered and subjected the Palestinian nations, including the Jews. Daniel and three other Hebrew youth were deported from the kingdom of Judah to Babylon to be instructed in the Chaldean language and culture, and to serve in the court of King Nebuchadnezzar. We find ourselves in the sixth century B.C. when Babylon, with its hanging gardens and other wonders, was one of the

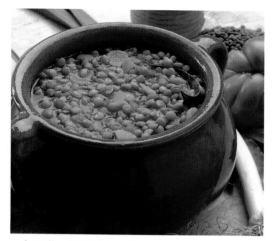

Lentils, together with other legumes, cereals and vegetables, were the food requested by the Hebrew youth deported to the court of King Nebuchadnezzar in the sixth century B.C., which is recorded as the first nutritional experiment in history.

richest and most flourishing powers in the ancient world. Let us enter the royal dining hall, where Daniel and his three companions were situated around the table, together with other Hebrews in exile:

"Pardon me, honorable Preceptor," says Daniel. "We cannot eat of these foods."

"What are you saying? These meats and wines are the most select, the best in Babylon! How dare you reject these delicacies? Don't you know that we are giving you the same food that His Majesty the King eats?"

"Yes, but we prefer to eat legumes and other vegetables, and have water to drink."

"You're crazy!" the Preceptor exclaimed. "I would be risking my position, and even my life, if the King came to know that because of not eating these meats you had become weakened and pale. I hope that you realize that I am responsible for your health!"

"All right", said Daniel. "We do not want to hurt you in any way. So, let's have an experiment. For ten days you will give us a vegetarian diet, and at the end of that time you look us over. According to the result, you yourself will make the decision. Is that all right with you?"

The Preceptor accepted the suggestion, sure that those strange but brave young men would not survive the test. But the text says[1] *"And at the end of ten days their countenances appeared fairer and fatter in flesh than all the children which did eat the portion of the king's meat."* And adds further, that from that moment on, the Preceptor gave them legumes and vegetables.

These young Hebrews were protagonists six centuries before Christ of one of the first practical demonstration which history records on behalf of a vegetarian diet. Their example has inspired many other young people of all times, like Daniel and his companions, to prefer to follow a simple vegetarian diet.

The results of a vegetarian diet continue to be as favorable today, or even more so, than they were in the time of the Neo-Babylonian Empire. There is no lack of examples of athletes, thinkers, and entire peoples who, following the vegetarian diet, reach high productive levels both physically and mentally. Furthermore, studies carried on in recent years (see pages 109-113) give greater credibility to that first experiment in nutrition recorded in the Biblical book of Daniel.

The Ancient Greeks and Romans

The nutritional habits of nations pass through well-defined stages. When a nation is struggling to become strong, its diet normally is frugal and consists mainly of foods derived from plants. As it becomes more prosperous, foods proceeding from animals are added. Later habits are formed of self-indulgence, gluttony and overeating. Historians and philosophers of all ages, on noting this tendency, have come to the conclusion that it is the cause of the fall of nations and empires. History has shown that when a nation reaches the zenith of its conquests, it is followed by another people with a simpler lifestyle, including also its nutritional habits.

Although they were not strict vegetarians, the Greek philosophers Pythagoras, Socrates, and Plato recommended a diet based on plant foods as a part of a program of natural life and hygiene. They opposed the use of meat because they believed that animal sacrifice was not noble, and that it abased the human spirit.

Citizens of the Roman Empire paid no attention to their wise men and philosophers, and entered a program of accommodation, gluttony and orgies, which ended with the fall of that great empire at the hands of the barbarians in the fifth century A. D. During the Middle Ages vegetarianism was practically ignored. Only some monastic orders followed a healthful and frugal diet.

The European Nations

During the Renaissance (sixteenth century) there was a renewed interest in classic Greek culture. As they studied the writing of Pythagoras, Hippocrates and other Greek wise men, some philosophers, artists and scientists such as Leonardo da Vinci and Andrea Vesalio discovered the value of plant foods in nutrition. Nevertheless, these ideas were known and followed only by a cultured minority. The great majority of the population followed a very poor and monotonous diet in which meat and sausages were the most appreciated foods, though they were not available for daily use.

At the close of the eighteenth century and the first years of the nineteenth, the

---

1. Daniel 1:15.

In the Golden Age when fruit
was the food,

nobody dared to contaminate
the mouth with bloody meat.

Then birds could move through
space with security,

and timid rabbits could run
safely through the brush;

and fish didn't need fear the
deceitful hooks.

There was tranquility for all, and
peace was real.

OVID
Latin poet, 1st century B.C.

first vegetarian societies were organized in England. There was a social movement which was concerned with the diet, brought on possibly by the unhealthful life and deficient diet of inhabitants in crowded urban areas created by the industrial revolution. These English movements on behalf of a healthful diet were exported to the colonies of the British Empire, especially to North America, where they took hold and developed with special intensity.

North America

William Metcalfe, was an English clergyman who in 1817 emigrated to North America. Landing in Philadelphia with 41 of his followers, Metcalfe gave the greatest impulse to the vegetarian movement in the New World. **Sylvester Graham,** a young Presbyterian minister, was one of his first disciples. Graham passed into the history of the human diet for having promoted the use of whole wheat flour, and for having practiced an original method of leavening dough. The well-known **Graham crackers** have perpetuated his memory.

Dr. Kellogg, Pioneer of Health Reform

Another one of the leaders in the flourishing movement on behalf of nutrition and a healthful lifestyle, which developed during the latter half of the nineteenth century, was **John H. Kellogg.** Under the sponsorship of the Seventh-day Adventist Church, in **Battle Creek** (Michigan), Dr. Kellogg established and directed one of the first and most important sanitariums in the western world of that time, where such revolutionary methods of treatment as a vegetarian diet, hydrotherapy, massages, and sun baths were applied. We should remember that in the middle of the nineteenth century, physicians still continued to apply heroic methods based on the theory of Galen's humors, with very little scientific basis, such as purging or blood-letting, and prescribing mercury, strychnine and other poisonous drugs. Little or nothing was known about the importance of a healthful diet, of physiotherapy, hygiene and preventive medicine in general.

Around the Seventh-day Adventist Battle Creek Sanitarium, pioneer of scientifically based natural remedies, both in the prevention and treatment of diseases, appeared the well-known Kellogg food industry, led by William, a brother of Dr. John Harvey Kellogg. Today, after the passage of almost a century, the breakfast based on whole-grain cereals is called the **"Kellogg Breakfast."**

A Woman Becomes the Leader

Among the pioneers of health reform which began in the United States during the middle of the nineteenth century, the name of a woman, **Ellen G. White,** stands out. With little formal education, during her long life she wrote over 100,000 pages, many of them related to health and diet, which still continue to be published in our day in many languages.

In 1863, when very little was known about the decisive influence of diet in the prevention of diseases, and much less about

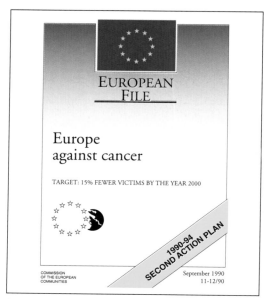

Increasing the consumption of fruit, vegetables and whole cereals, while reducing the intake of fats, is one of the ten points which constitute the European Code Against Cancer.

the importance of cholesterol and fats in heart diseases (coronary arteriosclerosis and heart attacks) **Ellen G. White** insistently recommended a diet based on plants (fruit, cereals and vegetables), in which there were no animal fats. She proposed the use of olive oil instead of butter, and a very moderate use of whole milk and eggs.

When she gave these warnings over a hundred years ago, few were ready to accept such dietary reforms. Actually, at that time no scientific reason was known for putting them into effect. But during the middle of the twentieth century, the great increase in cardiovascular diseases which was beginning to take place in the developed countries got scientists searching for the causes in the field of nutrition. And so in the middle of the 60's the conclusion was reached that the cholesterol found in animal fats (meat, sausages,

butter, eggs yolks) was the main cause of arteriosclerosis (hardening and narrowing of the arteries), together with other factors such as smoking, lack of physical exercise, and stress.

The whole world today is concerned about cholesterol, and many products include a label that says, *"No cholesterol."* When it is remembered that only animal products contain cholesterol, and that no plant food has it, it becomes clear that the vegetarian diet Mrs. White proposed presents many benefits for the prevention of heart attacks and other circulatory diseases. In the central and northern European countries where the use of butter is traditionally abundant, health authorities are promoting campaigns to encourage the populace to curb their use of butter, replacing it with vegetable oils. So the excess *"mountain of butter"* in Central Europe is causing serious problems to the European Community authorities, who do not know how to dispose of it. In the same way non-fat milk products are preferred, that is, those with a lower quantity of animal fat (milk with less than 30 - 40 grams of fat per liter), and a further recommendation that the use of refined sugar and sweets should not be abused, just as Ellen G. White proposed over one hundred years ago.

Another subject in which this pioneer in health education revealed a special understanding was the relationship between diet and cancer. She recommended a reduction in the use of meat and an increase in the use of plant foods (fruits, cereals and vegetables), as a way of preventing cancer. Very few listened to these counsels. But today, as we have said, the European Code Against Cancer counsels, among other things, the abundant use of fruit, vegetables and cereals with a high fiber content. Nobody today recommends the use of more meat, but rather suggest that its use be decreased, and that plant foods be substituted. The relationship between the intake of meat and cancer of the colon, among others, has been well demonstrated.

At present all medical and sanitary organizations recommend a reduction in the intake of animal products, and an increase in the use of fruits, whole grains, and vegetables, such as was proposed over a century ago by pioneers of health reform in North America.

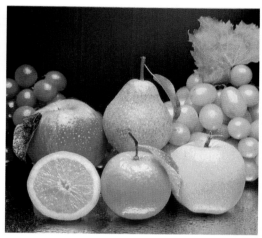

On March 4, 1993, the prestigious medical journal *New England Journal of Medicine,* published the results of research carried on by doctor ***Joan Sabate,*** of the School of Public Health of Loma Linda University (California). The report states that the habitual use of nuts, aside from providing a good amount of vegetable proteins and fats of great biological value, diminish the blood cholesterol level. In 1905 Ellen G. White had already said that nuts such as walnuts, almonds, etc. could well take the place of meat, and recommended their regular use. Up to quite recently these were thought of as a complementary item, to "snack" on at the time of gatherings and cocktail parties, without any great dietary value.

The teachings of this notable woman provided momentum to the vegetarian movement and health reform which was initiated in the United States around 130 years ago. Hers was one of the first voices to point out the perils of tobacco, when no one suspected that it could provoke cancer and was even prescribed by doctors. The same could be said of the use of drugs and alcoholic beverages.

Society owes a great debt of gratitude and recognition to these pioneers of public health. They had set as the objective of their reform to ensure the highest possible development of the body, mind, and spirit for the good of humanity. And they were successful. Their teachings are still a required point of reference for all those who are concerned with the health and well-being of individuals and communities, and are followed, both consciously or unconsciously, by millions of people throughout the world.

Conclusion

As we can see, there are many throughout history who have chosen a vegetarian diet, whether because of the health benefits, or for philosophical or religious motivation. To eat a diet based on fruit, cereals and vegetables is not a fad nor a radical idea, but a very ancient principle which has its origin in the creation of mankind.

Vegetarianism may be something new to some, but not to humanity which for millenniums has benefitted by it.

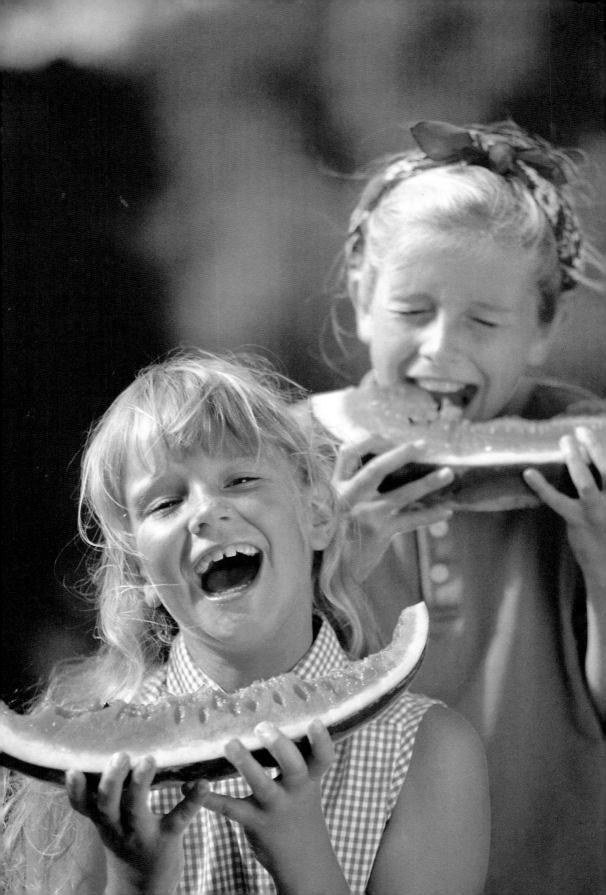

10

The Secret of Healthier Peoples

"T HE SICKEST sailors should stay on this island inhabited by Indians," said Captain Cartier. "Those who are in a better state of health will continue with me aboard ship, going toward the mouth of the St. Lawrence River."

That was the decision of **Jacques Cartier,** French navigator and discoverer, who had left the coasts of Europe around three months earlier. His purpose was the exploration of Canada, going up the St. Lawrence River. It was 1534, when scurvy, whose cause was unknown, was doing great harm among sailors who dared to cross the ocean. On the high seas they were fed with dried meats, sausages, wheat and fish. The lack of fresh foods, of fruit and vegetables during these long crossings, caused the travellers to sicken and die of scurvy caused by the lack of vitamin C (see page 73).

When Cartier made the decision of leaving a part of his crew on that island inhabit-

The degree
of strength
of a people depends
mainly on the nature
of its food.

HERBERT SPENCER
British philosopher
1820-1903

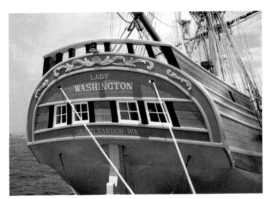

From the sixteenth to the eighteenth centuries, the lack of fruit and fresh vegetables in the diet of the navigators caused death to many of them because of scurvy, until it was discovered that just one lemon per day was enough to prevent that feared disease. Meat and eggs do not have vitamin C, and milk products have very little.

ed by Indians, 26 sailors had already died of scurvy during that part of the journey.

We are not acquainted with the motives that led Cartier to abandon his sick crew on an island inhabited by Indians, possibly hostile. Maybe he thought he was doing a favor to those poor sick sailors, allowing them to be buried on land—the last wish of every sailor—instead of being buried in the cold waters of the ocean. And possibly also his wish that his expedition be a success led him to abandon members of the crew who were suffering *"the complaint of navigators"* which could be a hindrance on the journey. Seen in this light, it was a painful but necessary decision.

"We will pass by and pick you up on our way home. May Providence protect you!" Captain Cartier shouted from his ship to the sick crew he had abandoned on the beach of that island.

Nevertheless the sailors who continued on the journey were sure that they would never see the sailors who remained on the island again, and that they would surely die very soon.

Some months later, on the return of the expedition up the St. Lawrence River, Cartier landed on that same island where he had left the sick sailors to die. The story had reserved for him a pleasing and instructive surprise:

They were all alive!

To his amazement, Cartier and his crew found all of their companions strong and healthy. They had been charitably fed by the inhabitants of the island with foods natural to that place: fresh fruit, vegetables and other plant foods; the ideal diet against scurvy! The simple and natural diet of the Indians restored health and vigor to those sturdy sailors who had become sick with scurvy as a result of a diet based on meat and fish, which, though sufficient in proteins and calories, was lacking in vitamins and other nutritive qualities which are found only in plant foods.

There are many examples, both in history and in present times, of primitive peoples who, following a simple diet based on plant foods, have enjoyed great vitality and longevity.

But is there any scientific evidence for the advantages of a meatless diet? What is the state of health of vegetarian peoples in light of present science?

The Inhabitants of Okinawa

Inhabitants of the island of Okinawa base their diet on plants (cereals, fruits and vegetables). Their longevity and fertility, as well as the absence of degenerative diseases, especially cancer, have drawn the attention of researchers.

During World War II, a group of military doctors performed a series of autopsies upon natives of the island who died in the conflict. They were able to see that even in persons of advanced age there were no tumors, no signs of arteriosclerosis (hardening of the arteries), neither arthritis nor other degenerative diseases.[1]

The Hunzas of Central Asia

The valley of Hunza is located in the north of Pakistan, near the border with China, and is surrounded by some of the highest and most massive mountains on earth: the Hindu Kush and the Karakorum. It is crossed by rivers, tributaries of the great Indus River, which form very deep valleys. The sides of the mountains have been terraced by the inhabitants so that grains and fruits, especially apricots, can be grown.

This is a remote area, enigmatic and legendary, because of the great longevity of its inhabitants. Its geographical isolation has permitted the survival of very healthful and natural habits of life, possibly for several millenniums.

The longevity and excellent health of the inhabitants of the valley of Hunza has drawn the attention of various researchers. For a long time it was thought that this extraordinary longevity was due only to genetic factors. But the interesting research carried on among this people has demonstrated that environmental factors play a much more important role than genetics. These are: a basically vegetarian diet, a sunny and dry climate, an austere lifestyle, and much physical exercise.

Doctors **Toomey** and **White,** outstanding North American cardiologists, visited this region in 1964 and carried on various studies which were published in the *American Heart Journal*.[2] They declared that the Hunzas maintained a very limited diet, based on fresh and dried fruits, nuts, different kinds of vegetables and cereals (barley, wheat and millet). They use some goat milk and eat lamb meat only once or twice a year, when they have feasts.

After studying 25 men who were between 90 and 110 years of age, these doctors came to the conclusion that they all had normal blood pressure, cholesterol and electrocardiograms. Cancer, heart diseases, diabetes or premature aging were unknown among the Hunzas.

Unfortunately the health of the Hunzas has changed within the last few years, for the "benefits" of civilization have reached them: canned foods, sweets, and industrially processed refined foods. The first cases of caries and digestive illnesses have appeared, unknown before this time. But in spite of all, they continue to be one of the most long-lived peoples on earth.

The *Sherpas* of Nepal

The *sherpas,* inhabitants of the rugged heights of the Himalayas, are famous for their extraordinary physical vitality. All expeditions to Mount Everest and other mountains of the region, depend on a group of *sherpa* porters. **Tenzing Norgay,** the sherpa who accompanied the English mountaineer **Sir Edmund Hillary** in the first ascent in history of Mount Everest, says in his autobiography *Tigers of the Snows:*[3] "Potatoes are our main crops, and are the basis of the sherpa diet, just as rice is for the Hindu and Chinese peoples. The varieties of potatoes which grow in the Himalayas are cultivated in lands found at a very high altitude (4,500 meters), which thus guarantees a supply of food in remote areas.

"Other basic foods in our diet are barley (which grows in an altitude up to 4,000 me-

continues on page 108

---

1. STEINER, P.E., Necropsies on Okinawans. Anatomic and pathologic observations. *Archives of Pathology*, **42**: 359 (1946).

2. TOOMEY, E. G.; WHITE, P. W. A brief survey of the health of aged Hunzas. *American Heart Journal*, **68**: 842 (1964).

3. NORGAY, T.; ULLMAN, J. R. *Tigers of the Snows*. New York, G. P. Putnam's Sons, 1955, page 14.

The Legendary

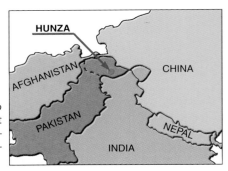

The Valley of Hunza is nestled between two massive mountain ranges, among the highest in the world: the Hindu Kush and the Karakorum in central Asia. Politically, it is a part of Pakistan. Its inhabitants are mostly Moslem.

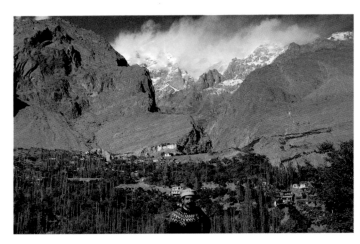

The Valley of Hunza is an enigmatic and fascinating region, both because of the magnificent scenery, as well as the **longevity** of its inhabitants.

In the terraces which have been built on the sides of the mountains, the inhabitants of the valley of Hunza cultivate **fruit trees** (above all, apricots) and **grains,** which are the basis of the diet of this long-lived people.

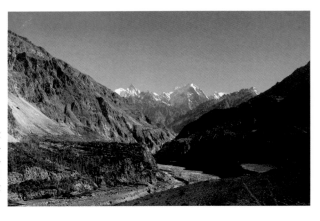

Valley of Hunza

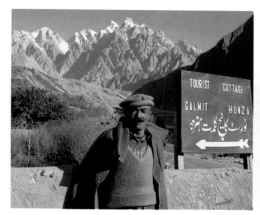

The access to the Hunza Valley is by a long and steep road that begins on the Pakistani city of Islamabad.

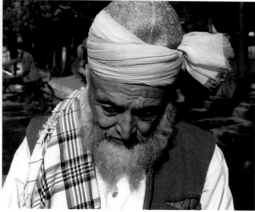

One of the many venerable centenarians of the Valley of Hunza, who at the age of 105 still carries on an active life.

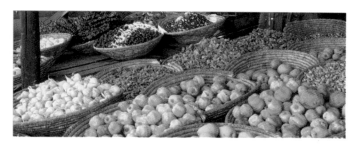

There is an abundance of high quality, excellent tasting **fruits, nuts** and **grains** in the stalls of the markets in the Valley of Hunza.

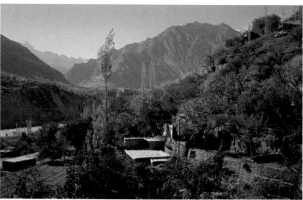

A basically vegetarian diet, physical exercise, a tranquil life and pure air seem to be the **secret of longevity** of the inhabitants of the Valley of Hunza, according to research which has been carried on.

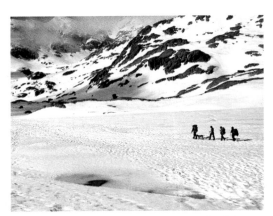

With a basically vegetarian diet, the "sherpas" of Nepal derive strength and physical vitality which have made them irreplaceable in all the expeditions to the Himalayas.

continues from page 105

ters) and wheat (up to 3,000 meters). The *sherpas* get milk and cheese from their flocks of sheep, goats and yaks with which they supplement their diet based on potatoes and cereals. Meat is hardly used, and the sherpas who are Buddhists are total vegetarians."

Otomi Indians

Otomi Indians live in the highlands of central Mexico, and their basic food is based on plants: corn"tortillas", beans, and different kinds of vegetables. Studies on this people, which were published in the *American Journal of Public Health*,[4] reveal that these people enjoy uncommonly good health. Cases of obesity, arterial hypertension or cancer are very rare or non-existent.

The British

Various studies were carried on in Great Britain during the decade 1970-1980, to see whether those who followed a vegetarian diet ingested enough calcium, and had bones that were sufficiently mineralized. The results surprised the researchers: the lactovegetarians had a higher percentage of calcium in their diet than the omnivorous, and their bones contained a larger quantity of this mineral.[5] As they age, vegetarians do not lose the calcium in their bones, while the omnivores suffer a progressive loss of calcium in their bones, causing them to soften.

The Seventh-day Adventists

One group that has aroused much interest among researchers is the membership of the Seventh-day Adventist Church, found scattered throughout the world in 204 countries. Adventists in general follow an ovolactovegetarian diet (some are strict vegetarians, without eggs or milk products) rich in fruit, whole cereals and vegetables. Furthermore they carry on a healthful lifestyle, with no tobacco, alcoholic beverages or other drugs. Seventh-day Adventists have been following this lifestyle for over one hundred years, with outstanding results.

The effects of this lifestyle are so striking because of their better health and greater longevity, that they have attracted the attention of investigators throughout the world. Some of the most prestigious scientific journals have published studies on the health of Seventh-day Adventists (see list of the main articles on page 112).

At the present time over 250 research studies have been reported on about this singular group of the population, composed of people of different races and cultures. In all

4. ANDERSON, R.K.; CALVO, J.; ROBINSON, W.D. *American Journal of Public Health,* **38:** 1126 (1948).

5. ELLIS, F.R.; HOLESH, S.; ELLIS, J.W. Incidence of osteoporosis in vegetarians and omnivores. *American Journal of Clinical Nutrition,* **25:** 555 (1972).

of these studies it has been demonstrated that Seventh-day Adventists enjoy better health than the rest of the population:

- **_Fewer_ heart attacks** (around 45% less than the general population).

- **_Fewer_** cases of **cancer,** both of the lungs (which can be explained by their abstinence of the use of tobacco), and the stomach or the colon (which may be directly related to a diet with very little or no meat). Seventh-day Adventists have fewer cases of breast, prostate or other organ cancers which have no direct relationship to dietary habits.

This reveals that a preventive action in diet and lifestyle exerts an influence upon the entire body, and not only on one specific organ. This interesting fact has attracted the attention of specialists in epidemiology and public health throughout the world. So much so that prestigious organizations such as the National Institute of Health of the United States are investing millions of dollars to study the health of the Seventh-day Adventist population. The interest of these official organizations in such studies, is to try to apply to the rest of the population the life habits and diet which have given Seventh-day Adventists such benefits.

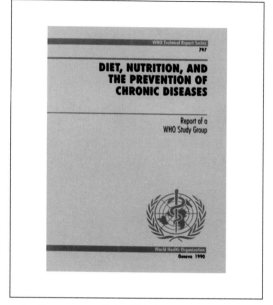

In the report of the World Health Organization, Diet, Nutrition and Prevention of Chronic Diseases, it stated that Seventh-day Adventists on different occasions have received special notice because of their low number of heart attacks, cancer and other diseases related to their lifestyle.

On What Are They Based?

Many researchers have asked, _What is the basis for Seventh-day Adventists to have adopted this healthful lifestyle? What motivation has led them to this?_

In first place, they start from the base that, just as **Moses** reported in the book of Genesis, God created the human being vegetarian.[6] **Cereals** and **fruit** were the first foods provided for the human race.

The diet which God provided mankind in the beginning must be the one that is best adapted to our needs, say the Adventists. And this reasoning does not seem to be faulty, for such prestigious institutions as the European Community recommend that "_fruit, greens and fresh vegetables and cereals with a high content of fiber_" be eaten (see page 100). As further research in the field of nutrition is carried on, it becomes more clear that there is a need of returning to a vegetarian diet based on fruit, cereals, and vegetables.

This kind of diet is exactly the one that is recommended at present to prevent diseases which cause higher mortality in western countries: heart diseases and cancer.

Furthermore, anatomical studies confirm the fact that the digestive system of a human

---

6. Genesis 1:29.

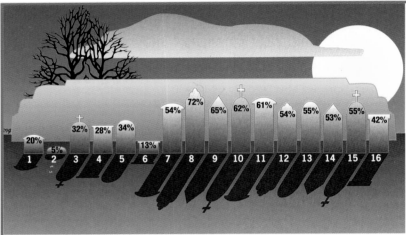

1. Lung cancer
2. Throat cancer
3. Bronchitis and emphysema
4. Cancer of the bladder
5. Cancer of the esophagus
6. Cirrhosis of the liver
7. Traffic accidents
8. Breast cancer
9. Cancer of the digestive tract
10. Leukemia
11. Evarian cancer
12. Cancer of the uterus
13. Heart attacks and angina pectoris
14. Cancer of the uterus
15. Diabetes
16. Gastroduodenal ulcer

Mortality among Seventh-day Adventists in comparison to the rest of the population

The figures show the percentage of risk of Seventh-day Adventists for each disease in relation to non-Adventists. Pages 112-113 give the bibliographical sources for these studies.

These figures have been obtained through an ample investigation conducted in California (USA) in which the cause of death of 27,530 Seventh-day Adventists was analyzed. The significance of these figures is as follows: For each 13 Adventists who died as the result of cirrhosis of the liver in this group, this same disease caused the death of 100 in another equal group of 27,530 non-Adventists.

It can be seen that the risk of cancer and heart diseases is significantly lower among Seventh-day Adventists when compared with the rest of the population.

being is more similar to that of the herbivorous animals, than the carnivorous. Mankind has been designed basically, from the anatomical and physiological point of view, to eat plant foods, although its adaptability also allows him to eat and assimilate meat (see page 126).

In second place, Seventh-day Adventists hold to that declaration of the apostle Paul which says, *"What? know ye not that your **body** is the **temple of the Holy Ghost** which is in you, which ye have of God, and ye are not your own? For ye are bought with a price: therefore glorify God in your body, and in your spirit, which are God's."*[7]

As believers, they do not consider their bodies to be the result of casual evolution; they are not their own but are a gift of God. They are persuaded that they have the duty of caring for and respecting their bodies as the supreme and marvelous work of a creating and loving God.

Seventh-day Adventists clearly understand that good health is not the result of happenstance, but comes from respect for the natural laws that God has given, and which we know through the study of human anatomy and physiology.

In third place, Seventh-day Adventists are a people who have **hope.** This in itself is a reason for good health. As a foundation for

---

7. I Corinthians 6:19-20.

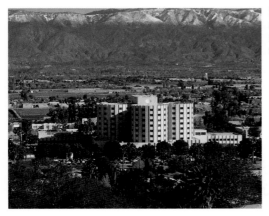

Loma Linda University, School of Medicine and Hospital, in California, USA, which belongs to Seventh-day Adventists.

Many people and social groups for various reasons and motives, have come to the conclusion that a diet based on plant foods is the healthiest and most satisfactory to the human being.

In the developed countries of the West, where the flesh diet has such deep roots, there is an increasing interest for the diet based on plant foods. Habits, health and science tend to increasingly agree among themselves every day.

their health they have the promise of the coming of "*new heavens and a new earth, wherein dwelleth righteousness*"[8] in which there will no more suffering nor pain, and where all mankind and nature will enjoy the splendor and beauty that they once possessed in the beginning.

In this glorious world, which is a common hope to all Christians, there will be no death, neither for individuals nor animals. There *"the wolf and the lamb shall feed together, and the lion shall eat straw like the bullock."*[9] No being will have to suffer and die so that another may live. The diet will be vegetarian for all, even those animals which are carnivorous. All will become as it was in the beginning.

One believer said, "The Bible shows how the human being began as a vegetarian, and at the end will be the same when everything is renewed. In the meantime, why not put into practice that which is ideal for mankind, as well as for all nature combined?"

In addition to being an internationally recognized high technology medical center, Loma Linda University also conducts studies concerning health care and a healthful lifestyle.

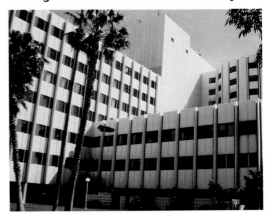

---

8. II Peter 3:13.
9. Isaiah 65:25.

Longevity of Seventh-day Adventists

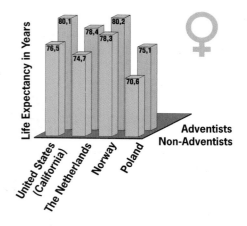

In the various studies carried on in the United States, the Netherlands, Norway and Poland, it has been observed that the expectation of life among Adventist women is between two and five years higher than the rest of the population, according to countries.

In the case of men, differences between Adventists and the general population are even greater, possibly due to a lower occurrence of heart attacks and other heart problems, which increases life expectancy among Adventists between four and ten years.

From the socio-health point of view these results are very exciting, and have awakened the interest of investigators throughout the entire world as well as of international organizations such as the WHO, because of the lifestyle of Seventh-day Adventists.

Some of the publications in which the results of the research are described are listed below in this page.

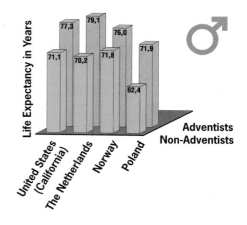

Some Scientific Publications Concerning the Health of Seventh-day Adventists

PHILIPS, R.L. Cancer among Seventh-day Adventists. *Journal of Environmental Pathology and Toxicology*, **3:** 157-169 (1980).

SCHULTZ, T.D.; LEKLEM, J.E. Dietary status of Seventh-day Adventists and nonvegetarian. *Journal of the American Dietetic Association*, **83:** 27-33 (1983).

BERKEL, J.; DEWAARD F. Mortality pattern and life expectancy of Seventh-day Adventists in the Netherlands. *International Journal of Epidemiology*, **12:** 455-459 (1983).

KAHN, H.A.; PHILIPS, R.L.; SNOWDON, D.A.; CHOI, W. Association between reported diet and all-cause mortality. Twenty-one-year follow-up on 27.530 adult Seventh-day Adventists. *American Journal of Epidemiology*, **119:** 775-787 (1984).

SNOWDON, D.A.; PHILIPS, R.L.; FRASER, G.E. Meat consumption and fatal ischemic heart disease. *Preventive Medecine*, **13:** 490-500 (1984).

SNOWDON, D.A.; PHILIPS, R.L. Does a vegetarian diet reduce the occurrence of diabetes?. *American Journal of Public Health*, **75:** 507-512 (1985).

FONNEBO, V. The Tromso heart study: Coronary risk factors in Seventh-day Adventists. *American Journal of Epidemiology*, **122:** 789-793 (1985).

JEDRYCHOWSKI, W. *et al.* Survival rates among Seventh-day Adventists compared with the general population in Poland. *Scandinavian Journal Society of Medecine*, **23:** 49-52 (1985).

MILLS, P.K.; ANNEGERS J.F.; PHILIPS, R.L. Animal product consumption and subsequent fatal breast cancer among Seventh-day Adventists. *American Journal of Epidemiology*, **127:** 440-453 (1988).

Relation Between the Consumption of Meat and the Relative Risk of Death from Certain Diseases

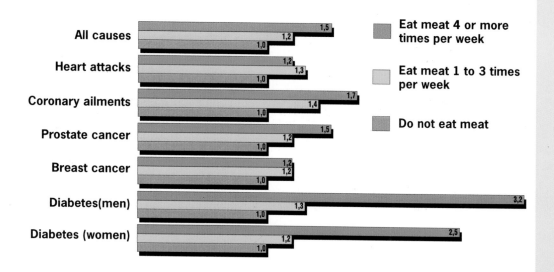

The figures reveal the risk of death for certain diseases in relation to the consumption of meat. As the latter increases, there is an increase of mortality for various reasons, especially of diabetes.

It is interesting to observe that these figures refer only to Seventh-day Adventists. None of them smoked or used alcoholic beverages, and their style of life was very similar, except in the kind of diet followed. If other factors do not intervene, this demonstrates that the differences between the Adventists who eat meat and the vegetarian ones can be almost completely attributed to their diet habits.

Bibliographical sources for this study are found below in this same page.

FRASER, G.E. Determinants of ischemic heart disease in Seventh-day Adventists: a review. *American Journal of Clinical Nutrition*, **48**: 833-836 (1988).

MILLS, P.K.; BEESON, W.L.; PHILLIPS, R.L.; FRASER, G.E. Cohort study of diet, lifestyle, and prostate cancer in Adventist men. *Cancer*, **64**: 598-604 (1989)

FRASER, G.E.; PHILLIPS, R.L.; BEESON, W.L. Hypertension, anti-hypertensive medication and risk of renal carcinoma in California Seventh-day Adventists. *International Journal of Epidemiology*, **19**: 832-838 (1990).

FRASER, G.E.; BEESON, W.L.; PHILLIPS, R.L. Diet and lung cancer in California Seventh-day Adventists. *American Journal of Epidemiology*, **133**: 683-693 (1991).

LINDSTED, K.; TONSTAD, S.; KUZMA, J.W. Body mass index and patterns of mortality among Seventh-day Adventist men. *International Journal of Obesity*, **15**: 397-406 (1991).

FONNEBO, V. Mortality in Norwegian Seventh-day Adventists 1962-1986. *Journal of Clinical Epidemiology*, **45**: 157-167 (1992).

GIEM, P.; BEESON, W.L.; FRASER, G.E. The incidence of dementia and intake of animal products: Preliminary findings from the Adventist Health Study. *Neuroepidemiology*, **12**: 28-36 (1993).

MILLS, P.K.; BEESON, W.L.; PHILLIPS, R.L.; FRASER, G.E. Cancer incidence among California Seventh-day Adventists, 1976-1982. *American Journal of Clinical Nutrition*, **59** (5 Suppl): 1136S-1142S (1994).

MELBY, C.L.; TOOHEY, M.L.; CEBRICK, J. Blood pressure and blood lipids among vegetarian, semivegetarian, and non-vegetarian African Americans. *American Journal of Clinical Nutrition*, **59**: 103-109 (1994).

KUCZMARSKI, R.J.; ANDERSON, J.J.; KOCH, G.G. Correlates of blood pressure in Seventh-day Adventist (SDA) and non-SDA adolescents. *Journal of the American College of Nutrition*, **13**: 165-173 (1994).

FRASER, G.E.; LINDSTED, K.D.; BEESON, W.L. Effect of risk factor values on lifetime risk of and age at first coronary event. The Adventist Health Study. *American Journal of Epidemiology*, **142**: 746-758 (1995).

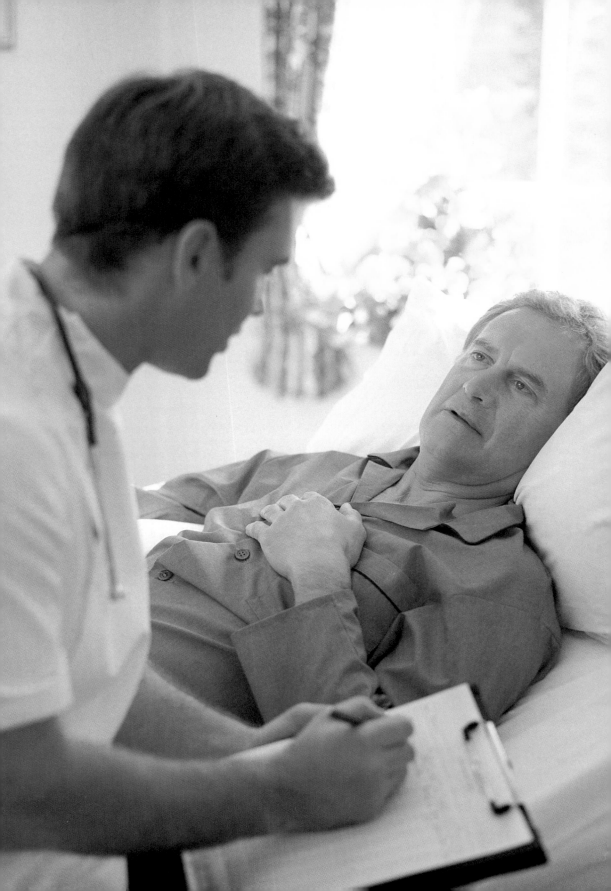

Good Reasons for Change

W E ARE now living in a period of resurging interest in vegetarianism as never before in the past. But different from other times, when the defenders of a vegetarian diet were experienced mature men within the environment of philosophy and science, today it is the youth who are searching with such enthusiasm for a more simple and natural lifestyle.

Such famous universities as Yale, in the United States, offer their students a menu which includes whole and ecological vegetarian foods. Hamburgers and other meat products with French fries, which for years was the favorite food of young people in developed countries, are being replaced by products based on soybeans, whole cereals prepared in various ways, salads, and garden products which have been biologically grown, without preservatives, coloring or other additives.

Wisdom lies in the ability to discover an alternative.

BERNARD JENSEN
Contemporary physician

Motives for Health

Up until the decade of the 1970's experts in nutrition were more concerned with dietary deficiencies—wanting people to eat sufficient calories—than worried about the quality of the foods. It was during the first half of the twentieth century that the myth about proteins was reaffirmed. More proteins should be consumed (more than were really necessary) and the best way of doing this was to turn to meat products.

But during recent years researchers and experts in nutrition have concluded that the quality of foods is more important than the quantity; that the need for proteins are less than was thought (see page 59), and that the nutritional problem of developed countries is precisely the excess intake of animal foods, fats and sugar, and the lack of plant products (fruits, cereals and vegetables).

More recently there have been more and more declarations in favor of the vegetarian diet, both by researchers and preventive medicine experts, and by official institutions and organizations, national and international. Recommendations are not heard via the media that people should eat more meat. Instead there is an insistence on the need of ingesting an abundant amount of vegetables.

The **American Dietetic Association,** recognized by its well-balanced declarations, stated in 1980 that *"there is more and more scientific evidence which supports a positive relationship between a diet based on plant foods and the prevention of certain degenerative chronic diseases such as obesity, coronary diseases, arterial hypertension, diabetes, cancer of the colon, and others."*[1]

In Spain, Professor **Grande Covián,** one of the foremost authorities in nutrition in his country, in spite of his criticism of vegetarianism, says in his book *Nutrición y salud,* *"The ovolactovegetarian diet can actually be perfectly satisfactory from the nutritional point of view."* And he finally recognizes that *"even the strict vegetarian diet may be adequate for adults if consideration is given to correct its evident limitations,"* and that *"meat is not indispensable for the nutrition of mankind."*[2]

Doctor **Miguel Aguilar,** associate in the Spanish Royal Society of Physics, and researcher for the Superior Council of Scientific Investigations, in his work *La dieta vegetariana: un camino hacia la nutrition equilibrada,*[3] demonstrates by scientific arguments that the **vegetarian diet** is generally **superior** to the **omnivorous** and the **western diet** in particular. In this interesting publication, there is demonstrated, with the strength of statistics, the numerous "clichés" that western society has in relation to meat: that its proteins are of a superior quality, or that it is the best source of iron.

Cardiovascular Diseases

In the interesting report published recently by the **World Health Organization** (WHO), *Diet, Nutrition and the Prevention of Chronic Diseases,* there is a section dedicated to cardiovascular diseases in which an international group of experts has gathered

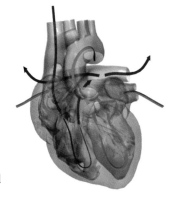

1. *Journal of the American Dietetic Association,* **77**: 61 (1980).
2. Grande Covián, F. *Nutrición y salud.* Madrid, Ediciones Temas de Hoy, 1990, pages 26, 39.
3. Aguilar, M. *La dieta vegetariana.* Madrid, Ediciones Temas de Hoy, 1990, page 251.

research related to the advantages of a diet based on plant foods. One paragraph says:

The population subgroups which consume diets rich in plant foods, present lower rates for coronary cardiopathy than the general population. For example, the rates on cardiopathy among the Seventh-day Adventists in Norway and the Netherlands are equivalent to one-third or one half of those observed in the general population. Seventh-day Adventists who eat meat have higher rates than the vegetarians, and British vegetarians have a mortality rate for coronary cardiopathy 30% lower than that found among non-vegetarians, even taking into consideration a lower consumption of cigarettes. Concentrations of cholesterol are much lower than those found among ovolactovegetarians and the non-vegetarians.[4]

Kahn, Philips and other researchers[5] (see references on page 112) published a study conducted at **Loma Linda University** (California) with 27,530 Seventh-day Adventists, of which half were ovolactovegetarians or strict vegetarians. The results revealed that coronary deaths (myocardial attacks) among Adventists happened only 55% as often as the rest of the population. And more: Adventists who ate meat more than four times per week run the risk of having

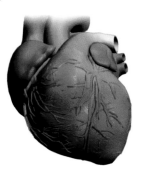

70% more deaths as a result of coronary diseases (factor 1.7) than vegetarian Adventists (see page 113). Inasmuch as none of them smoke, and all follow a similar lifestyle, the differences in the risk of having a heart attack are due solely to nutrition.[6]

In the prestigious medical periodical *Lancet*, a recent study of those affected by arteriosclerosis showed that 82% of those who followed a vegetarian diet low in fats, abstained from tobacco, and carried on a program of physical exercise, were rewarded with a lowering of the cholesterol deposits which narrow the arteries and make difficult the passage of blood.[7]

Cholesterol

A strict vegetarian diet has no cholesterol, since this substance is found only in animal foods. No fruit, cereal or vegetable contains cholesterol. The body is able to produce its own needed cholesterol, beginning with fatty acids in the diet. But when, in addition, large quantities of cholesterol are taken in with foods, its level in the blood increases dangerously (see page 49).

Vegetarians have a lower level of cholesterol in the blood, which protects them against the development of arteriosclerosis, heart attacks, cerebral thrombosis and other cardiocirculatory problems. It has been demonstrated that vegetarian Seventh-day Adventists have an average level of 149 mg/dl of cholesterol, while non-Adventists who eat meat have an average of 214 mg/dl.[8] A study was done in Australia aimed at demonstrating the effect of diet upon cho-

4. WHO, Technical Report Series, No. 797, (*Diet, Nutrition, and the Prevention of Chronic Diseases*). Report of a WHO Study Group. Geneva, World Health Organization, 1990, pages 62, 63.

5. KAHN, H.A.; PHILIPS, R.L.; SNOWDON, D.A.; CHOI, W. Association between reported diet and all-cause mortality. Twenty-one-year follow-up on 27.530 adult Seventh-day Adventists. *American Journal of Epidemiology*, **119**: 775-787 (1984).

6. PHILIPS, R.L. Cancer among Seventh-day Adventists. *Journal of Environmental Pathology and Toxicology*, **3**: 157-169 (1980).

7. *Lancet*, **336**: 129-133, 1990.

8. *American Journal of Clinical Nutrition*, **40**: 921-926 (1984).

lesterol levels. One group of individuals was given to eat, among other things, 250 grams of lean meat each day, while another group was given the same diet, but substituting the meat with gluten and soybean proteins. After six weeks, vegetarians lowered their cholesterol level twice as much as those who followed the lean meat diet.[9]

Cancer

For various reasons the vegetarian diet protects against cancer:

* It is *rich in* substances which pro- tect against cancer which are only found in plant food: carotene or provitamin A (carrots, bell peppers and other brightly-colored vegetables), enzymes which in-activate carcinogenic benzopyrene (in cabbage and lettuce)[10] inhibitors of pro- teose (in legumes) and antioxidants (vita-min C).

* It contains *abundant* vegetable fiber, whose absence increases the risk of can-cer of the colon. Meat contains no veg-etable fiber (cellulose). Fiber absorbs and flushes the carcinogenic substances that may be in the intestines, and does the same with cholesterol and biliary salts.[11]

* Normally vegetarians consume *much less* fats than non-vegetarians. Fur-thermore, vegetable fats generally con-tain mono or polyunsaturated fatty acids, with a protective action against cancer and favoring health. It has been demonstrated that as the intake of ani-mal fats increases, the mortality from breast cancer rises.[12]

* A diet based on vegetables is *exempt from carcinogenic substances* which are found in **meat,** nitrites and hormones to fatten cattle.

In a report of a group of **WHO** experts, *Diet, Nutrition and Prevention of Chronic Dis-eases,* it was indicated that "*the lower rates of colon and rectal cancer among Seventh-day Adventists in California (where several studies have been conducted on this subject) half of which are vegetarians, support the hypothesis of a protective effect in vegetarian diets, al-though this portion of the population also ab-stains from alcoholic beverages*".[13]

As previously mentioned (see page 100), the *European Code Against Cancer,*

9. *American Journal of Clinical Nutrition,* **50:** 280-287 (1989).

10. *Committee on Diet, Nutrition and Cancer, National Research Council, EE. UU.: Diet, Nutrition, and Cancer,* Washington, Na-tional Academy Press, 1982.

11. PAGE, H.S., ASIRE, A. J. *Cancer rates and risks,* Bethesda, National Cancer Institute, 1985.

12. CARROLL K. K. *Dietary polyunsaturated fat versus saturated fat in relation to mamary carcinogenesis. Lipids* **14:** 155-158 (1979).

13. WHO, Technical Report Series, No. 797, (*Diet, Nutrition, and the Prevention of Chronic Diseases*). Report of a WHO Study Group. Geneva, World Health Organization, 1990, page 70.

coinciding with what has already been presented, recommends a diet based on fruits and fresh vegetables, as well as whole cereals rich in fiber, or whole grains.

Obesity

Most of the studies that have been conducted generally show that those whose diet is based on plant foods, weigh an average of four to ten kilos less than those who eat meat habitually.[14]

According to the report of a group of WHO experts,[15] there is more proof that demonstrates that an excess of fat in the diet favors a weight increase. The greater the proportion of calories coming from fats, the greater the risk of obesity.

These statistical reports and experiments, published in the report of the WHO, agree that vegetarians ingest a lower quantity of fats, both in absolute terms (grams of fat per day) and relative (see page 48 on the proportion of calories which should be derived from fats).

Blood Pressure

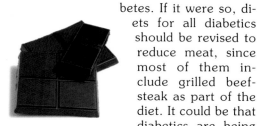

According to the report of WHO experts, *the epidemiological studies systematically indicate that blood pres-*

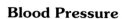
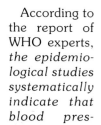

sure among vegetarians is lower than among non-vegetarians (...) Though it is not easy to determine the exact cause for these results, the studies point out that some component of the products originating with animals, possibly the proteins or fats, may affect blood pressure among well-fed peoples.[16]

The report also recommends that in order to avoid hypertension and obesity, a diet low in fats and high in complex carbohydrates (for example, whole cereals), should be followed, and reduce to a minimum the ingestion of alcohol and the use of salt.

Diabetes

Those who do not eat meat run a lower risk of suffering diabetes. Furthermore, some studies suggest that the habitual and abundant use of meat could be related to the cause of diabetes. If it were so, diets for all diabetics should be revised to reduce meat, since most of them include grilled beefsteak as part of the diet. It could be that diabetics are being recommended that which aggravates their disease. However, the diets of all diabetics have been revised in the past 20 years to reduce animal fat and increase use of complex carbohydrates.

continues on page 121

---

14. *Journal of Human Nutrition,* **35:** 437 (1981); *New England Journal of Medecine,* **292:** 1148 (1975); *Journal of the American Dietetic Association,* **77:** 655 (1980).

15. WHO, Technical Report Series, No. 797, (*Diet, Nutrition, and the Prevention of Chronic Diseases*). Report of a WHO Study Group. Geneva, World Health Organization, 1990, page 79.

16. *Ibíd,* page 67.

Physical Endurance According to Diet

A Diet of Fats and Proteins

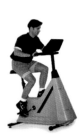 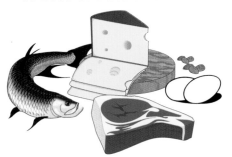

The results of the experiment executed in Sweden* indicate that athletes who eat a meat diet rich in fats and proteins are the first to become tired when they carry on a sustained effort.

Time of continued pedalling of a bicycle: **57** minutes

A Mixed Diet

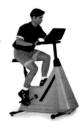 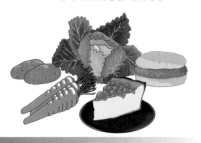

With a mixed diet including both animal and plant foods, the resistance to fatigue as measured by a continuous pedalling of a bicycle, increases up to 114 minutes.

Time of continued pedalling of a bicycle: **114** minutes

A Vegetable Diet Rich in Carbohydrates

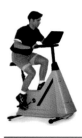 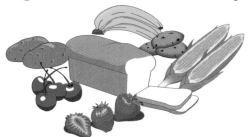

The best results for guaranteeing resistance are obtained by athletes whose diet is based on foods rich in carbohydrates, especially cereals (grains) and fruits.

Time of continued pedalling on a bicycle: **167** minutes

* SCHARFFENBERG, JOHN. Why be a vegetarian? Life and Health supplement, 1: 14 (1973).

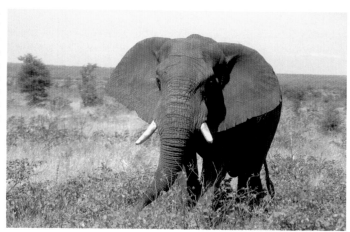

Herbivorous animals show greater capacity for physical resistance than carnivorous. The rhinoceros and the elephant, both herbivorous, are probably the strongest animals known.

continues from page 119

Osteoporosis

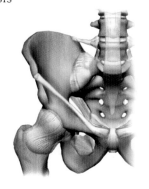

Ovolactovegetarian women generally have less osteoporosis than those who habitually eat meat.[17] Osteoporosis within recent times has become a disease which concerns women more after menopause. It consists of the loss of mass and consistency of the bones, which makes them susceptible to fractures and deformation (see page 85).

Researchers are investigating the reason why women who follow an ovolactovegetarian diet suffer less osteoporosis than those who eat meat, while in both diets the consumption of calcium is the same. But it is thought that, by a mechanism which is still not well known, the intake of a large amount of protein in the diet based on meat causes the organism to eliminate more calcium through the urine.[18]

Physical Endurance

It is a known fact that physical endurance against fatigue of vegetarian athletes is superior to that of those who indulge in a meat diet. Those who eat a lot of meat have more "starting power" to reach maximum strength in a short time, but they tire more quickly. This is the case with weight lifters who have a high protein diet derived from much meat. They are capable of extraordinary strength at a given moment, but they lack endurance.

The same can be said of animals. How is it possible that a deer can escape the chase of a lion? Simply because a lion develops greater speed at the beginning of the race, but if it is not able to reach its vegetarian victim, the latter tires the lion right away. The endurance of herbivorous animals is much greater. And not only the endurance: The

---

17. *Journal of the American Dietetic Association,* **76:** 148 (1980).
18. *Nutrition Action,* june 1982.

rhinoceros is one of the animals which develops a greater pushing power, and is strictly a vegetarian. The elephant, the buffalo and the ox are other examples of vegetarian animals with great muscular endurance and proverbial strength.

Swedish investigators carried on an experiment with well-trained athletes, having them pedal a stationary bicycle. After following a diet rich in animal products, with abundant proteins and fats for three days, they reached a maximum time of pedalling without stopping of 57 minutes (average time). During the next three days they partook of a mixed diet (meat, milk, potatoes, vegetables and fruit) and the average pedalling time rose to 114 minutes. But after following a vegetarian diet, rich in whole cereals and nuts, as well as fruits, legumes and vegetables they reached an average 167 minutes of continuous pedalling![19]

Ethical Motives

There are persons who have reached the conclusion that they should follow a vegetarian diet (fruit, cereals and vegetables) for ethical reasons. Evidently, these cannot be measured nor analyzed with scientific criteria, and each one is free to assume them or not. In this field all of us must exercise a great amount of tolerance—which is so much needed by humanity today—respecting the opinions and beliefs of others.

The Respect of Life

The respect for the life of animals as a reason for not eating meat is a very ancient idea. Oriental religions such as Buddhism, show great kindness and compassion for animals, although there are those who relate this more with the transmigration of the soul (any animal may be the bearer of a human soul) than respect for the animal itself. Anyway, it is certain that there are many people in the Far East who from ancient times have avoided killing animals for food. This idea was also developed in classical Greece and Rome: Pythagoras, Porphirius and Ovid, among others, thought that killing animals for food contaminated and brutalized the human spirit. *"When will you make an end to these horrible killings?"* asked the Greek philosopher Empidocles in the fifth century B.C.

Throughout history there have been many artists, philosophers and scientists who have shared these sentiments about animals. Leonardo da Vinci, Gandhi, Edison, Bernard Shaw, Rabindranath Tagore and Tolstoy were vegetarians. It is enough to see how a child becomes fond of a chicken or any other domestic animal to realize that sacrificing an animal to eat goes contrary to human nature.

Created to Suffer

Not only killing animals has raised moral questioning among different countries and peoples. The cruel and inconsiderate way in which many are cared for, transported and sacrificed, awakens a rejection in many. The professional periodical *El Médico* (The Physician) said in an article dedicated to modern techniques of animal production:

"Life in a cattle-raising locale is as follows: New-born calves are separated from their mothers. They are fed skimmed milk and spend the first months of their lives without moving, in stables with a temperature of 37 degrees Centigrade (= 98.6°F. In this way they drink more than a normal

---

19. SCHARFFENBERG, J. Why be a vegetarian? *Life and Health Supplement,* **1:** 14 (1973).

There are vegetarians who have become vegetarians for purely ethical reasons, based on respect for the life of animals. If those who eat meat had to personally sacrifice animals, there might be many more vegetarians.

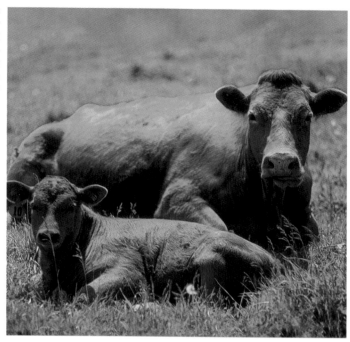

animal would ... and furthermore they eat a puree of proteins which more quickly develops the prized white meat. The objective of their existence—the slaughter house—is reached when they are swollen with antibiotics as a preventive measure, of beta-blocking substances against the permanent risk of heart attack, and sedatives against stress. "[20]

Respect for Human Life Itself

Ethical motives for abstaining from meat can also be presented in another aspect aside from respect for animals: respect for the body of the individual himself. This was understood by the pioneers of the movement in behalf of a healthful lifestyle that was developed in the United States in the middle of the nineteenth century (see page 99). Following ethical and religious principles, they

came to the conclusion that they should abstain from all that might harm the good operation of the organism: drugs, alcoholic beverages, tobacco, and unhealthful foods such as meat and its derivatives.

Today there are many throughout the world who, based on religion or otherwise, endeavor to apply the same ethical principles of healthful living and respect for the human body.

Ecological and Economic Motives

Raising animals for food is a luxury, an authentic waste from the economic point of view. If the large quantities of cereals and legumes used as food for farm animals, as well as land and water used to fatten these animals were dedicated to human consump-

---

20. *El Médico*, 28th October 1988, pages 74, 75.

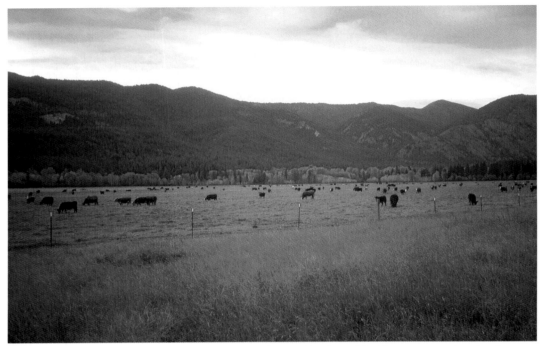

If the cereals and legumes dedicated to the production of fodder were used to feed human beings instead of feeding animals for meat production, hunger throughout the world could easily be eliminated.

tion, hunger throughout the world could easily be eradicated. For each 5,000 calories in the form of corn (1.4 kilos) which are used to feed a cow, only 200 calories are recovered in the form of meat (130 grams). An inhabitant of the third world could be fed several days with these 1.4 kilos of corn, but 130 grams of meat is barely sufficient for one beefsteak on the table of a western inhabitant. The production of meat requires great quantities of grain only for the feeding of cattle.

If 100 square meters of soybeans are planted, around five kilos of proteins will be obtained, with which the needs of 70 persons can be covered for one day. But if these five kilos are used to feed cattle, only one-half kilo of meat will result, which will barely cover the daily protein needs of only two persons.

Solidarity Against Hunger

There are citizens sensitive to the unbalanced nutritives of the inhabitants of our planet who find in these figures an important reason for abstaining from animal foods. Poor countries are forced to sell to the rich, so that they may feed animals, grain and soybeans which really are needed by their own inhabitants. **Solidarity,** to which so many recur to fight hunger throughout the world, could be obtained by simply assigning

A vegetarian diet is more economical than a meat diet. Based on the same nutritive principles, meat is more expensive than legumes.

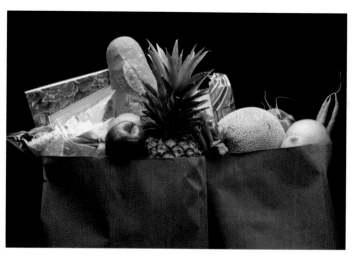

for human consumption the thousands of tons of cereals and soybeans which are used to feed cattle. This would imply that those who live in rich countries reduce their ingestion of meat (which, furthermore, would improve their health) and increase the use of cereals and legumes. And if the eating of meat were left off completely, there would be no problem from the nutritive standpoint, for it has been more than demonstrated and accepted by all the experts that **meat *is not*** an **indispensable** component of the human diet.

We are not dealing with utopia. The nutritive quality of soybean proteins is equal to or surpasses that of meat, and products made from soybeans and grains may be more attractive and tasty, as we can see in businesses which specialize in health foods.

The Market Basket

Economic reasons may also be important to an individual. All nutritive reasons being the same, **meat** is ***more expensive*** than legumes, cereals or potatoes. In a study carried on in the United States in 1990, it was calculated that a diet based on a low amount of saturated fats and cholesterol, with little meat and few dairy products, would save the consumer 230 dollars per year.[21] So the **vegetarian diet** is not only ***more* healthful,** but furthermore is ***less* expensive.**

21. *Circulation* **81:** 1721-1733 (1980).

Is Mankind Designed To Eat Meat?

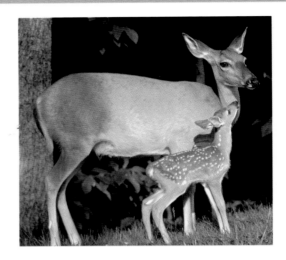

Herbivorous animals have a digestive system similar to that of human beings.

From the time of the Renaissance anatomists have been interested in comparing the **digestive system** of animals with that of man. "To what kind of mammals is the human being most similar—the herbivorous or the carnivores? Let us rapidly review the main characteristics of the kind of digestive organs in man and animals:

Teeth

- **Carnivores:** Prominent fangs which can cut and tear meat, barely chewing it.
- **Herbivores:** Well-developed molars which allow for chewing food until it becomes a paste.
- **Man:** Human teeth are small, different from those of the carnivores. The molars are more similar to those of herbivores, able to chew and tear into pieces vegetable fiber and cereal grains.

Jaws

- **Carnivores:** Only allows for the movement of opening and closing to tear the food.

- **Herbivores:** Allows for lateral movement to tear and salivate the foods, as well as opening and closing.
- **Man:** Can perform all kinds of movement with the jaws, as the herbivores.

Saliva

- **Carnivores:** Has an **acid** reaction (low pH) necessary for the digestion of meat proteins.
- **Herbivores:** Has an **alkaline** reaction (high pH) permitting better digestion of carbohydrates.
- **Man:** Saliva is **alkaline,** as that of the herbivores. It further contains **ptyalin** and **amylase,** enzymes which initiate the digestion of starches which are found only in vegetable foods. It is therefore a saliva appropriate for eating vegetable foods.

Intestines

- **Carnivores:** Its digestive track is much **shorter** than that of the herbivores. The reason for this is that meat has to be digested and eliminated rapidly, for its decomposition and putrefaction in the intestines produces harmful substances that poison the animal.

- **Herbivores:** Have a **very long** digestive tract which permits a relatively slow movement of foods (up to three days). Vegetable foods need a long time for digestion, but do not putrefy in the intestines neither do they produce toxic substances. If a herbivore ate meat, it would become intoxicated, for having to retain the food in the food for such a long time to travel the full length, it undergoes putrefaction with the consequent liberation of toxic materials.

- **Man:** His intestines are proportionally **longer** than the carnivores, though not as long as the herbivores. For this reason he can eat meat, though there is the possibility that he may suffer the process of putrefaction, especially when there is constipation and slow transit. Thus toxic substances are liberated (**cadaverines** and **indole,** among others) which are passed on to the blood and produce headaches, allergies, eruptions and many other symptoms.

As a whole, we can see that the digestive system of man is more similar to the one of herbivorous animals than of the carnivorous. Nevertheless although man's digestive organs are planned basically for biting, chewing, and digesting plant foods, they have a great capacity for adaptation, not existent in animals, permitting man to eat practically anything.

So we can say that the **human being is anatomically and physiologically a vegetarian,** although he has the possibility of adapting to an omnivorous diet.

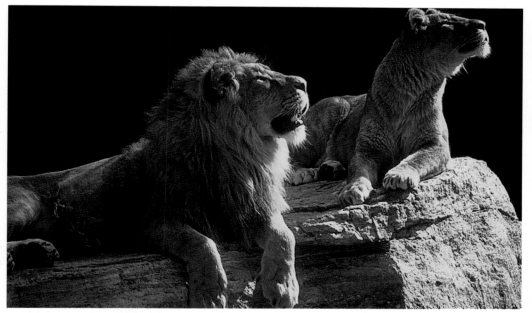

Carnivorous animals have much shorter intestines than the herbivorous, for meat must be digested and eliminated repidly to avoid the production of putrefaction and toxic substances (known as cadaverines). This is what generally happens in the human intestines, which are longer than those of carnivores (though not as much as the herbivores), causing headaches, cutaneous eruptions and allergies especially in the case of constipation.

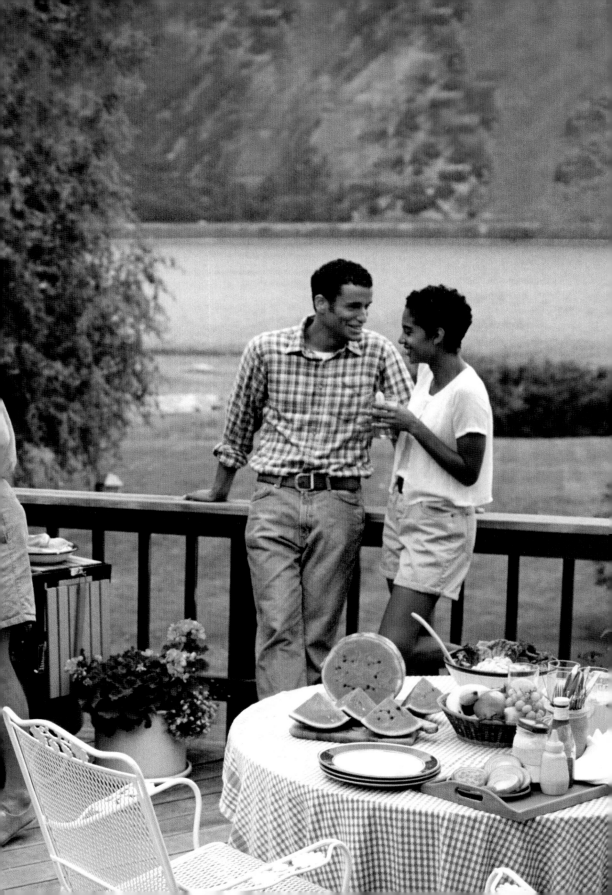

12

Problems With Meat

MEAT has never been a healthful food. Though eaten sporadically, as it happened prior to the industrial age, it did not cause many health problems. In *earlier times* the main repercussion on health caused by eating meat was the transmission of **infections** and **parasitosis.**

Nevertheless, eating meat at the present time has some other risks. The bacterial and parasitical contamination has diminished, thanks to the improvements made in the techniques of hygiene, although they are still present. The detrimental effects of meat which mostly concern consumers today in highly developed countries are those derived from intensive cattle raising on farms and industrialized exploitation: artificial **foods, hormones** for rapid fattening, **antibiotics, tranquilizers** against stress, *and a long list* of artificial chemical substances in an attempt to reduce the numerous diseases which animals suffer.

I am conscious of the fact that eating meat does not harmonize with the greatest wisdom.

ALBERT SCHWEITZER
Physician and winner
of the Nobel Prize for Peace
1875-1965

All this, combined with the unnatural conditions surrounding the breeding of cattle, only increases the problems of most meats available in today's market, even though producers may guarantee that they do not contain pathogenic microorganisms.

Traditionally meat was eaten on specific occasions coinciding with the slaughter of animals or with feasts, and during the rest of the year meat eating was sporadic. At the present time meat is available at any supermarket every day of the year, therefore it can be eaten daily, if so desired. In ancient times this was only within reach of the rich.

Unnatural breeding methods for meat, combined with its permanent availability, mean that meat consumption carries with it considerable risks which should not be ignored.

An Excess of Saturated Fatty Acids and Cholesterol

Meat has a high proportion of fats most of which are formed by saturated fatty acids. Due to the sedentary conditions of the animals that are bred in modern cattle corrals, which reach almost total immobility, the meat, though it looks lean, contains much fat. This happens in the case of pork, for example: its lean meat contains around 18% fat.

The excess of **fats** in the meat diet and in products *originating from* **animals** is responsible, together with **tobacco, stress,** and **sedentary** habits, for the increase of **cholesterol** in the blood. This substance is deposited on the arterial walls, hardening them and narrowing the passageway, a process which is known as **arteriosclerosis.** This narrowing of the arteries is the basic cause of myocardial **attacks,** cerebral **thrombosis** (stroke), and *the lack* of **blood flow** in the extremities.

Food originating with animals produce an increase of cholesterol in the blood in two ways:

Fat content
in some types of meats

Part of the animal	Grams of fat for each 100 grams of edible food
PORK	
Bacon	57.5
Carcass	35.1
Salami	33.7
Ham chopped, canned	18.8
Loin	12.6
Cure Ham	8.3
LAMB	
Retail cuts, lean and fat	21.6
Leg of lamb	17.1
Retail cuts, lean	5.25
BEEF	
Veal, loin	9.14
Veal, sirloin	7.8
Retail cuts, lean and fat	6.8
Veal, leg	3.1
Retail cuts, lean	2.9
FOWL	
Duck	5.95
Quail	4.53
Chicken	3.1
Turkey	2.86

The figures refer to raw meat.

- Because they **contain cholesterol** which is absorbed into the intestines and pass directly into the blood (see the table on page 49). Plant foods have no cholesterol.

- Because they **contain** a *large quantity* of **saturated fatty acids** which increase the production of cholesterol in the body itself. Vegetable foods contain mostly unsaturated fatty acids which regulate or lower the level of blood cholesterol.

A diet rich in meat and its fatty derivatives, such as sausages, as well as in shell fish, is a very important cause in the increase of cholesterol and in the appearance of **arteriosclerosis**. Other foods that originate with animals (eggs, cream, cheese) also contribute to this.

There are clear indications that the risk of getting certain kinds of **cancer** is directly connected to the amount of total fats in the diet.[1] This gives another reason for reducing the intake of fats. The WHO recommends that the ingestion of saturated fats vary between 0% (that is, nothing) and 10% of the maximum calories in the diet (see page 48). At present, in most of western countries, fats represent up to 45% of the total ingested calories, with a high proportion of saturated animal fats. Countries which have initiated an educational campaign to lower fat intake such as the US have now reduced it to 34% of total calories. The more meats and foods that are derived from animals as a part of the diet, the more risk there is of suffering from arteriosclerosis, cancer, obesity and other diseases.

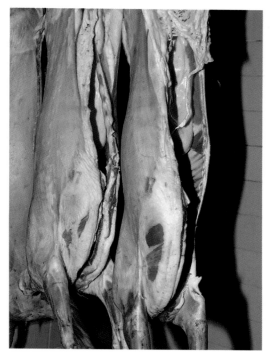

Even meat that looks lean contains a large proportion of fat, due to the sedentary and artificial life conditions of the animals in the industrial exploitation of cattle.

Cancer

Did you know that one kilo of grilled beefsteak has as much **benzopyrene** (a cancer producing agent) as 600 cigarettes?[2] The cancerous effect of benzopyrene has been well demonstrated. Consumption of well-done meat by barbecuing, or grilling has been associated with an increased risk of colon, stomach and esophaegal cancer.[3]

1. WILLETT, W.C. *et al.* Relation of meat, fat, and fiber intake to the risk of colon cancer in a prospective study among women. *New England Journal of Medicine,* 23: 1664-1672 (1990).
2. LIJINSKY, W.; SHUBIK, P. Benzopyrene and other polynuclear hydrocarbons in charcoal-boiled meat. *Science,* **145:** 53-55 (1964).
3. WARD, M.H. *et al.* Risk of adenocarcinoma of the stomach and esophagus with meat cooking method and doneness preference. *International Journal of Cancer,* **71:** 14-19 (1997).

Importance of Diet in Stomach Cancer

"It has been demonstrated that diet is the principal factor in the etiology of **gastric adenocarcinoma** (stomach cancer)." So began an article published recently in a Spanish weekly medical journal. It emphasizes the fact that this type of cancer is one of those which results in more deaths per year throughout the world. It has been proven that an excessive consumption of **salt** leads to an increase of bacteria in the stomach. These act by transforming food **nitrates** (used widely in the meat industry) into **nitrites,** which when combined with the **amines** and **urea** present in the digestive tract, produce **nitrosamines** and **nitrosureas,** which are recognized as being carcinogenic.

Stomach cancer is related to the abundant use of **smoked** and highly **seasoned** meat and fish. This has been demonstrated in Japan where the customary diet contains many foods of this kind, and where stomach cancer is very frequent. Another cause that is being investigated is the lack of certain vitamins which play an extensive protective role against cancer.

- **Vitamin A** in its provitamin form (carotene): **inhibits** the formation of **free radicals** which play an important function in the formation of malignant tumors.

- **Vitamin C** (can only be found in plant foods): Among many other activities, it has the one of **thwarting** the transformation of **nitrates** into **nitrites** and nitrosamenase.

- **Vitamin E:** It acts as an **antioxidant,** which protects cells from degenerative changes.

The **reduction** in the use of **salt, nitrates,** as well as **smoked** products, combined with an **increased** use of **fruits** and **fresh vegetables** in the diet, is the **best way of avoiding stomach cancer,** according to current knowledge.

Although you may not eat grilled meat, you still will not be free of ingesting carcinogenic substances. **Methylcolantrene** is one of these substances formed when meat is heated to a high temperatures as it is fried or grilled. When methylcolantrene is given in large quantities to laboratory animals, they develop cancer. But methylcolantrene, even when given in small quantities, though it does not result directly in cancer, sensitizes the animals that eat it. When these enter into contact with some other carcinogenic agent, even though it may be in a small quantity, they develop a malignant tumor. We may say that the methylcolantrene found in meat adds *strength* to the action of other **carcinogenic** substances which all of us may take in at one time or another.

Often cattle which are found in slaughter houses, when cut apart reveal some kind of **tumors,** whether benign or cancerous. Generally this is cut out ... but not always. But what happens to the rest of the animal? It is certain that some cancerous cells remain

Pork is the meat that has most fat. Some of its derivatives such as York ham (cooked ham) has as much as 40% fat, for which reason it is strongly unadvised for the health, in spite of the custom—fortunately becoming less frequent—of giving it to the sick.

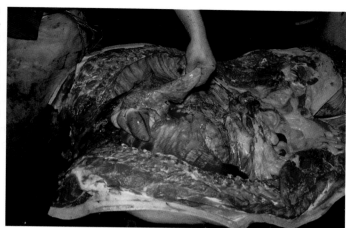

An Anti-Cancer Diet

According to the report of a WHO study group, it has been demonstrated that the diet which provides the least risk of suffering from certain types of cancer such as the colon, prostate, breast, stomach and esophagus, is this:

- Content **low in** total and saturated **fats.**

- Content **high in plant origin foods**, especially green, yellow and red vegetables, as well as citric fruits (oranges, tangerines, lemons, etc.)

- **Low content in alcohol; cured, smoked and pickled foods.**

* WHO, Technical Report Series, No. 797, (*Diet, Nutrition, and the Prevention of Chronic Diseases: Report of a WHO*). Study Group. Geneva, World Health Organization, 1990, page 74.

in the lymphatic glands, in the blood, or in other organs. In the 1960's studies were carried out which demonstrated the transmissibility of certain types of cancer produced by viruses, among laboratory animals.[4]

Though it is true that there is no definite and conclusive proof that eating cancerous animal meat will produce cancer in human beings, there still are some indications of this, and investigation is being carried on at present along this line.

Be it as it may, research has demonstrated that the heaviest consumers of animal products (meat, milk, cheese and eggs) have a total risk of cancer 3.6 times greater than non-consumers.[5] A study was carried on at Harvard University covering 89,000 women

4. GRACE, J. T.; MIRAND, E. A.; MOUNT, D. T. Relationship of viruses to maignant disease. *Archives International Medicine*, **105:** 482-491 (1960).
5. SNOWDON, D. A.; PHILIPS, R. L.; CHOI, W. Diet, obesity, and risk of fatal prostate cancer. *American Journal of Epidemiology*, **120:** 224-250 (1984).

Scavengers of the Sea

Shell fish transmit the **hepatitis A** virus, the "Cholerae vibrio", a microorganism which causes **cholera,** and other pathogenic microorganisms. One out of four cases of **toxic infections** result from the eating of **clams** and other **small sea creatures.**

These are **natural purifiers** of the seas, for they filter the water, developing an ecological function similar to that done by vultures and other scavenger fowls on earth. These sea animals are **necrophagous,** that is, they feed on dead marine creatures. As a result they frequently are contaminated by a wide spread of pathogenic and toxic microorganisms. It is quite probable that much of the summer **gastroenteritis** which is blamed on the long-suffering mayonnaise is actually caused by the sea food which the mayonnaise frequently accompanies.

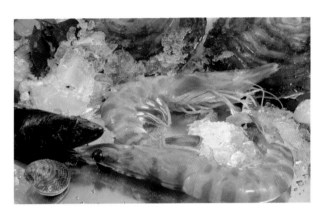

Besides this, sea food contains abundant **cholesterol,** produces **uric acid** and is **hard to digest.** Taking all into consideration, they are not a healthful food, despite the myth that surrounds them.

who were followed for six years, and the conclusion was reached that a larger consumption of red meats and animal fats increases the incidence of colon cancer.[6] Many others surveys have reached the same conclusion, for instance one performed in California.[7]

Parasitism

In some places of the world, trichinosis is so widely spread that the risk of contracting

it is reason enough not to eat pork or boar meat. In developed countries there still are cases of **trichinosis** which often result in death, especially for having eaten boar meat or pork which have not undergone sanitary inspection.[8]

Other Infections

Animals get sick as much or more than people. Year after year millions of dollars are lost because of animal diseases, especially

continues on page 136

6. *New England Journal of Medicine*, **323:** 1664-1672 (1990).
7. PROBST-HENSCH, N.M. Meat preparation and colorectal adenomas in a large sigmoidoscopy-based case-control study in California (United States). *Cancer Causes Control*, **8:** 175-183 (1997).
8. LANDRY, S.M. *et al.* Trichinosis: common source outbreak related to commercial pork. *Southern Medical Journal*, **85:** 428-429 (1992).

African Porcine Disease

The African swine pest is produced by a **DNA type virus** which only affects **pigs and boars.** Up to the present time, there is no effective vaccination or treatment for it. The only remedy is the destruction of the sick animals.
These are the kidneys of a pig that died of the porcine disease. They reveal edema, inflammation and ecchymosis (hemorrhaging).

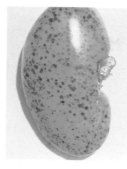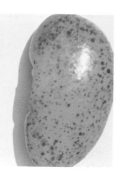

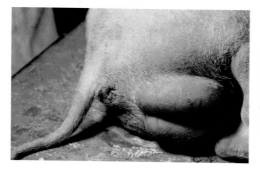

Orchitis (inflammation of the testicles) is one of the most characteristic lesions of the African swine disease. The meat of the infected animals contain up to 100,000 viruses per gram.
Although this virus does not affect man, the sale of infected meat is considered to be a fraud by authorities, because of its poor quality.

Inflamed intestinal glands, typical of pigs that have died as a result of the African swine disease. According to the Spanish Ministry of Agriculture, the trend of this disease has been downward in recent years. Nevertheless, out breaks of these and other diseases among pigs are very often around the world.

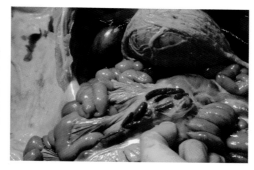

Foot and Mouth Disease

Foot and Mouth Disease is a highly contagious viral disease; possibly the most contagious of all those affecting animals. It particularly affects sheep, goats, cows, pigs and other animals with cloven hoofs. It appears with fever, blisters in the mouth and on the hoofs and myocarditis (inflammation of the cardiac muscle), which usually is the cause of death.

In spite of what is normally said, Foot and Mouth Disease is considered as a zoonosis, that is to say, a disease transmisible to human beings.* The symptoms in humans are similar to those that appear in animals (fever and blisters), although it is not usually serious according to data available at present. In most of the cases registered, the infection of people by animals has occurred due to a direct contact with infected animals.

According to official information, meat or milk from animals suffering from Foot and Mouth Diesease—which in principle should not enter the food chain, do not transmit the virus to humans. However, this disease weakens the animals and it must affect the quality of the food products obtained from them. Once more, this shows the deterioration in animal health that mass production of meat and milk entails.

* Foot and Mouth Disease: the human consequences. *British Medical Journal* 2001; **322:** 565-566.

An Animal With a Tendency Toward Disease

The pig is an animal with the tendency toward the transmission of diseases. Traditionally it was fed garbage (this is still a custom in rural areas), and through rats they acquired trichina and other parasites.

Modern cattle raising has improved the hygienic conditions, but other problems have been derived as a result of intensive breeding. Expecting a pig to reach the weight of 100 kilos (220 lb) within five or six months, or even before, makes it necessary to accelerate growth through artificial means. This, combined with the fact that the breeds used are highly selected (and are therefore very delicate), explains why animals have very small resistance to diseases and are victims of frequent epidemics.

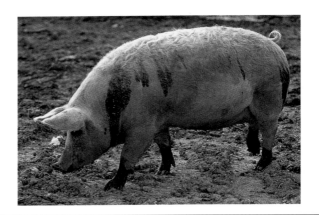

The **African porcine disease,** pseudorabies (which especially affects the male pigs), **atrophic rhinitis,** and parasitism such as **trichina,** are the most frequent diseases among swine.

continues from page 134

those of an infectious type. According to data supplied by the General Subsection of Animal Health of the Ministry of Agriculture [of Spain] in 1992, 65,184 cases of bovine tuberculosis were detected (2.13% of the controlled animals), and 148,557 of ovine brucellosis (Maltese fever), (2.41% of the controlled animals), among other infections. In all developed countries, cattle with positive skin tests for tuberculosis should be destroyed, but this is not always the case.

Many of these animal infections are treated with *large doses* of **antibiotics,** part of which remain in the **meat** that is eaten and are even passed to the **milk.** Even the **food** which is generally fed to the cattle contains small doses of antibiotics such as penicillin and tetracycline. Cattlemen in the United States were the ones who discovered, around thirty years ago, that animals who were fed with foods containing antibiotics, had less illnesses, developed better, and even grew faster.

Now then, risks to the health of those who eat meat have not been unnoticed: **Resistances, allergies** and **sensitivity** to antibiotics may be provoked, even unknowingly, by the use of meat from animals which have been fed or treated with them. And many allergic reactions of unknown cause are due to the eating of meat which contains the remnants of antibiotics and other allergizing substances.

The *massive use* of **antibiotics** in the breeding of animals is generating **bacteria resistant** to drugs. Various investigations indicate that commercially produced meat may be the way through which bacteria resistant to these antibiotics are transmitted to human beings, resulting in infections which are difficult to treat.[9] **Chicken** meat is the product which *most frequently is* **contaminated** with pathogenic microorganisms (**salmonella,** above all) as reported by the *Food and Drug Administration* of the United States (FDA).

Furthermore, meats may be of themselves carriers for the transmission of infections due to the facility with which pathogenic germs proliferate in them: salmonella, brucellosis (or Malta fever), tuberculosis and hepatitis, among many.

Hormones and Other Chemical Substances

Alarm has sounded throughout Spain, and other western european countries when in the 90's persons had to be hospitalized with symptoms of intoxication and hepatitis, all of them having eaten meat from animals coming from farms where they were fattened by **clembuterol.** This substance which gives meat a very reddish and healthy appearance is one of the hormonal derivatives whose use is forbidden by the European health authorities. But even the authorized substances are subject to revision and criticism by many experts who consider that their use in food animals has negative consequences upon the health of human beings.

For example **dietilestilbestrol** (DES) is used on chicken farms to produce chickens that are fattened 15% faster with 10% less feed. It is a derivative of estrogens (feminine hormones), which have a **cancerous** reaction upon human beings. In spite of the prohibition, it is suspected that they are still being used.

Ham (dry or sweet), sausages and almost all pork products are cured with **nitrate** and **sodium nitrate.** These substances, aside from avoiding putrefaction by anaerobic germs like those of the *Clostridium* type (which cause gangrene in human tissues), give meat a rose or red color which makes them more appetizing. But these nitrates and nitrites can be combined with amines in the human intestine, forming **nitrosamines,** which are strongly carcinogenic. The habitual use of foods containing nitrosamines produces cancer in experimental animals, and also in man.[10]

■ ■ ■

After analyzing these problems related to a meat diet, the question might be asked, *Why not substitute meat and its derivatives with foods that are more healthful?* You will find counsels on making this change in a progressive way on page 171.

---

9. *Journal of the American Medical Association,* **258:** 1496-1499 (1987).

10. POBEL, D. *et al.* Nitrosamine, nitrate and nitrite in relation to gastric cancer: a case-control study in Marseille, France. *European Journal of Epidemiology,* **11:** 67-73 (1995).

Mad Cow Disease

In spite of the fact that the number of people affected by the human variant of this disease is relatively low, great social anxiety has arisen throughout Europe. This is possibly due to the fact that it is a very enigmatic disease, with great uncertainty regarding how it is caught. Up to the present day **there is still no possible treatment.**

Definition: Bovine Spongiforme Encephalitis (BSE) is a degeneration of the brain tissue making it take on the aspect of a sponge. A type of abnormal protein called pathogenic **prion** causes it. In human beings spongiforme encephalitis caused by the consumption of meat products contaminated with prions is called the "new variant of the **Creutzfeldt-Jakob disease**".

Transmission method: It mainly affects mammals and it is transmitted from one to another when **they eat** parts from other affected animals. It is also transmitted through the **blood** (for example, transfusions) and possibly by the **skin** (there have been some cases of infection from beauty creams prepared using bovine derivatives).

Transmission sequence: Spongiforme encephalitis has been known about in sheep livestock for over two hundred years as scrapie.

- **Cows** became contaminated when they were fed mixed feed prepared using offal from ill sheep or goats, a practice that has been habitual over the past few decades in Western Europe.

- The **mixed feed** prepared using offal from cows, some of them ill, have been being used in Europe as food for other cows, therefore meaning that the disease has become widespread among cattle.

- **Human** are contaminated when they eat meat products made with SRM of ill animals, or when coming into contact with other contaminated products.

Course of the disease in humans: Between 5 and 15 years (or even more) after having eaten contaminated animal tissues or having had contact with them, the following symptoms appear: progressive memory loss, anxiety and depression, muscular spasms, impaired motor coordination and dementia. Death occurs several years after the symptoms have appeared.

SRM (Specific Risk Materials): this is the name for the parts of the animal that can transmit the disease when they are eaten by a human being or by another animal. They are the **brains,** the peripheral **nerves,** the bones (and **gelatin** that is prepared using them), the **viscera** (including the intestines) and the **blood.** Lean meat without bones or nerves does not seem to transmit the disease; neither does milk.

Prevention: As there **is not treatment,** those who wish to eat meat should **avoid eating** or coming into **contact with SRM** from contaminated animals.

13

A Balanced Diet

NO FOOD by itself can provide all the nutrients necessary for the body. For that reason, our diet should include a variety of products. The **pyramid of a healthful diet** (see page 141) shows in what **proportion** each of the different kinds of **food** should be found on our tables.

Group 1 Foods
Eat Abundantly

As can be seen on page 141, the **base** of our diet should be made up of foods from **Group 1: fruits, grains** (always whole, if possible) and **vegetables.** These foods can be and should be used in **great quantity,** as much as desired. The only limit affecting the quantity of fruit, cereals or vegetables that a person may eat daily is determined by

Grains (cereals), fruits, nuts and vegetables make up the food chosen for us by the Creator.

ELLEN G. WHITE
North American writer and educator
1827-1915

Recommended Daily Diet
(for adults)

Group 1

Cereals (including bread): 4 portions
- One ration of breakfast cereal (approximately 4-6 tablespoons)
- One cereal soup (one soup plate)
- Two slices of bread (one slice = approximately 100 grams)

Vegetables: 2 portions
- One salad (including carrots, peppers, tomatoes or any other colored vegetable)
- Two servings of boiled or baked vegetables (peas, spinach, artichokes, etc.)

Fresh fruit: 3 portions
One serving is a large fruit (apple, pear, orange, peach) or 200 grams of any fruit (cherries, strawberries, etc.)

Nuts: 1 portions (= one handful)

Group 2

Protein foods: 2 portions
One portion is a plate of legumes or a soy product, or one egg.

Milk products: 2 portions
One portion is a glass of cow or soy milk (200 ml) or a yogurt (125 ml) or 100 grams of cottage cheese or milk curd.

Group 3

Fats: 2 or 3 spoons olive or seed oil.

Children, adolescents, and pregnant or breast-feeding **women,** should increase the daily rations of milk and its derivatives. This may be soy milk provided it has been enriched with calcium and vitamin D, or provided that supplements are taken of both.

the total of **calories** that the individual must consume according to his activity (see page 160).

Fresh Fruits and Vegetables

Fruit and vegetables provide a good quantity of plant **fiber,** simple carbohydrates (**sugars**), and complex (**starch**) carbohydrates, **vitamins** and **minerals.** Fruit is the main source of **vitamin C,** especially citric fruits (oranges, lemons, grapefruit, etc.), kiwi and currants. All fruits contain **proteins** of great biological value, though in small quantities.

continues on page 142

A Pyramid of
a Balanced Diet

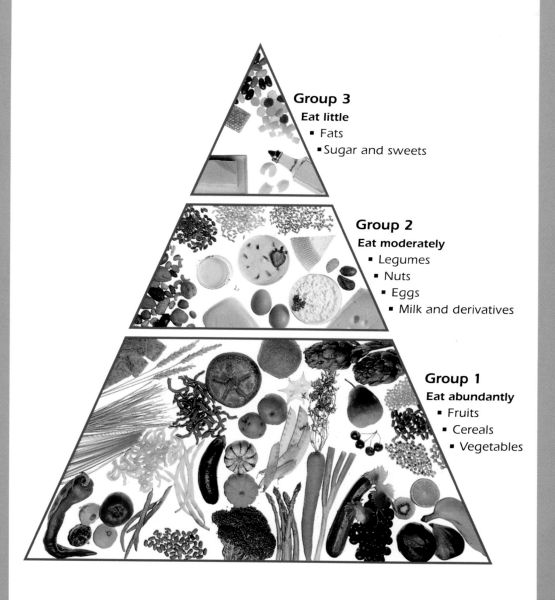

Group 3
Eat little
- Fats
- Sugar and sweets

Group 2
Eat moderately
- Legumes
- Nuts
- Eggs
- Milk and derivatives

Group 1
Eat abundantly
- Fruits
- Cereals
- Vegetables

The Incompatibles

In dealing with the food incompatibles, which seem to concern some, we must bear in mind the following physiological realities:

- Our bodies **need a variety of nutrients,** and they should be combined in a correct proportion.

- **Combining proteins** of different food elements is how we increase their biological value.

- For our bodies to take adequate advantage of the amino acids coming from different foods, these **should be eaten together in the same meal or within 6 to 8 hours.** Our bodies will get more good out of the proteins in rice and lentils if they are eaten in the same meal, than if they are eaten separately at different times.

- The different vitamins and minerals that our bodies need every day **are distributed unequally throughout the different foods.** Some contain more of certain vitamins, and others contain different vitamins. This is another reason for following a varied diet.

As we can see, mixing different kinds of food at the same meal is natural and necessary for a healthy person. There is no need to worry excessively whether certain foods are incompatible, to the point of referring to long tables, as some do, to know which foods may be eaten in combination. The following norms are sufficient:

- **Do not make excessive mixtures of foods** at the same meal, to avoid overloading the digestive system. The variety offered by a salad, two foods and a dessert needs not to be added with other foods.

- Each person should **avoid foods which cause digestive problems,** even when they are eaten alone. Many times what is called an incompatibility is actually an **individual intolerance** to a given food.

- **Every body is different.** There may be mixtures of foods which some cannot tolerate but others may enjoy. Each much study himself and then act wisely.

- There are a few combinations that generally produce **digestive upsets** to most of people: large amounts of fruits and vegetables in the same meal, milk and sugar (produces fermentation in the stomach), bread, pasta and potatoes; as well as the mixture of different kinds of fats.

continues from page 140

There are also vegetables which contain a fair amount of proteins when, for example, compared with meat which has 15 to 21 grams per 100 grams: potatoes (2 grams), artichoke (3 grams) or peas (5 grams) (see page 56).

Colored vegetables such as carrots, spinach, tomatoes and peppers have important quantities of **vitamin A** (carotene) which play a preventive part against the formation of malignant tumors, as has been demonstrated in experiments on animals.

Cereals (grains)

Grains are the food base in most of the world. Wheat, originating in the Mediterranean countries, has spread to all the temperate areas of the earth; rice in Asia; corn in the Americas; millet in Africa. Cereals are the main source of energy because of their *high content* of **complex carbohydrates,** or glucides.

Group 2 Foods
Eat moderately

Foods from Group 2 (see page 141) are those which contain an important proportion of **proteins,** such as **legumes, nuts, milk** and its derivatives, **fish** and **meat.** These foods should be eaten *in moderation,* that is, controlled quantities. We should not lean toward increasing the consumption of these foods, but rather decreasing them. Furthermore, within this group, we should tend to substitute meat and fish with plant foods. This change should take place gradually, following the guide listed on page 174.

The greatest need of proteins takes place during the **growth years.** The majority of adults who live in developed countries eat too much protein. There are still those who think that proteins of plant origin are of lesser quality. Nevertheless we now know that legumes such as **soybeans,** which provide **proteins** of *high biological quality,* can be compared to those of meat and milk, with *all* of the **essential amino acids.** Others, which are not complete of themselves (lentils, beans, chickpeas, etc.) are so when they are eaten with grains (rice, wheat, oats). The mixture of both kinds of foods (**legumes** and **cereals**) provide **complete proteins,** similar in quality to meat (see page 62).

Fruits and vegetables also have proteins, as we have said (see page 56), so that it is easy to supply the daily need for protein when a varied diet based on plant foods is eaten.

Group 3 Foods
Use Small Amounts

Fats

Fats of **animal origin** (butter, fatty cheese, pork, sausages) are among the *most harmful* elements in the western diet. They increase the **cholesterol** level and contribute to **arteriosclerosis** (hardening and narrowing of the arteries), which, together with cancer, cause the highest amount of deaths in developed countries. They are not a necessary part of the diet, and can be *very well* **substituted** with vegetable fats: olive, corn oil or soybean oil.

Sugar

Refined sugar is a source of calories, providing no other nutrient. For this reason it is said that sugar only offers *"empty calories."* On the other hand, fruits and grains contain unrefined sugars and complex carbohydrates, as well as vitamins, minerals and vegetable fiber.

A Pattern for a Daily Diet

As soon as you get up: drink one or two glasses of tepid or warm **water**—not cold. Cold water while fasting may provoke a disagreeable reaction on an empty stomach. On the contrary, warm water brings blood to the stomach in preparation for breakfast.

Breakfast

Should be rich in foods that supply **energy,** *especially* **carbohydrates** (glucides). It may be composed of all or some of the following foods:

- **Grains** (wheat, oats, barley, rye, etc.) In addition to bread (we recommend that it be whole grain), it is good to eat other cereals:

  ✓ In the form of breakfast cereals (which can be shared with fruit juice, milk or yogurt).

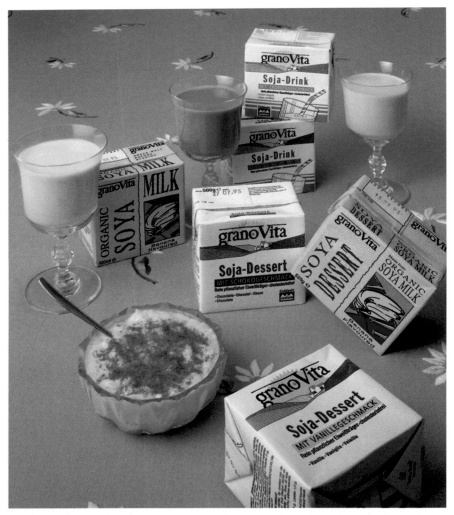

In markets today there are more and more soybean-based products, such as custards and other desserts. They have the advantage of being totally vegetable, and therefore have no cholesterol.

✓ In the form of flakes, cooked with milk, or with vegetable broth. Oatmeal cooked in milk for ten minutes is very nutritious, easily digested, and tasty, especially if a banana, raisins or apple slices are added.

• **Soy or cow milk** (skimmed for adults), yogurt, fresh cheese or cottage cheese (rich in proteins with the advantage that it has practically no fats). Those who want a totally vegetable breakfast may substitute milk products with the so-called vegetable milks, based on soybeans, or almonds.

Soybean milk can be compared to cow milk because of its richness in proteins

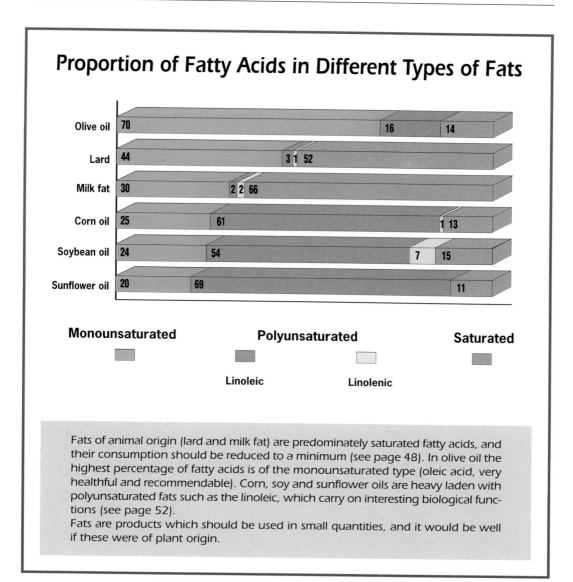

Proportion of Fatty Acids in Different Types of Fats

	Monounsaturated	Polyunsaturated		Saturated
		Linoleic	Linolenic	
Olive oil	70	16		14
Lard	44	3 1		52
Milk fat	30	2 2		66
Corn oil	25	61	1	13
Soybean oil	24	54	7	15
Sunflower oil	20	69		11

Fats of animal origin (lard and milk fat) are predominately saturated fatty acids, and their consumption should be reduced to a minimum (see page 48). In olive oil the highest percentage of fatty acids is of the monounsaturated type (oleic acid, very healthful and recommendable). Corn, soy and sunflower oils are heavy laden with polyunsaturated fats such as the linoleic, which carry on interesting biological functions (see page 52).

Fats are products which should be used in small quantities, and it would be well if these were of plant origin.

and other nutrients, being only less abundant in calcium and vitamins A, B_{12}, and D. Because of this, those who habitually use soy milk should search for other sources of calcium, especially children and pregnant women. Nevertheless you may find in the markets soy milk enriched with calcium, vitamins A and D, and even B_{12}, which makes it a complete food. Babies who are allergic to cow milk, and are fed exclusively with soy milk, testify to its nutritional value.

How to obtain an Ideal Breakfast

- Try to get up **15 - 20 minutes earlier** than usual.

- Reserve the most **appetizing foods** for breakfast.

- Think of breakfast as **another meal** that must be programmed and prepared.

- **Eat a light early supper,** or nothing.

- **Set the breakfast table** the previous night.

In oriental countries such as Japan, *tofu* is used extensively. This is a vegetable cheese based on soybeans. It is rich in proteins with the advantage that it has no cholesterol or animal fats.

- **Nuts** (almonds, walnuts, hazel nuts, peanuts, etc.) provide proteins, unsaturated fatty acids of high biological value (like the linoleic and the linolenic) and minerals (rich in calcium and iron). As has been demonstrated by **Dr. Joan Sabate** and other researchers at Loma Linda University, a handful of nuts contributes to lowering blood cholesterol (see page 101).

Young children, and those who do not have good health, may eat nuts ground up (i.e peanut or almond butter).

- **Dried fruits** (raisins, dried prunes, dried peaches, apricots, or others): They provide energy-giving natural sugars, and furthermore prevent constipation, especially the dried prunes.

- **Fresh fruits:** May be ingested in the form of juices, although the whole fruit is preferable because contains fiber. Have at least one citrus (orange, tangerine, grapefruit or lemon) per day. It is a good habit to eat one apple just at the beginning or end of breakfast. It combines well with all other foods, and is nutritive and easily digested.

- **Dietary complements:** Those who need a supplementary portion of nutrients may include some dietary complement in their breakfast. Breakfast is a good time to take these, for during the rest of the day the body can benefit from their strengthening effect. These may be taken dissolved in milk or fruit juice.

  ✓ **Wheat germ:** Provides large quantities of group B vitamins, as well as proteins and lipids containing essential fatty acids. It is rich in essential amino acids.

  ✓ **Brewer's yeast:** It is also rich in group B vitamins and in minerals. Additionally has a tonic effect upon the body.

  ✓ **Flower pollen:** Contains proteins and essential amino acids, as well as elements which stimulate resistance to infections.

  ✓ **Soy lecithin:** This is a phospholipid which performs notable functions in the body, especially upon the nervous system (an equalizer) and upon cholesterol (it lowers the level of cholesterol in the blood).

The Noon Meal

It should be made up of:

- **A salad of fresh vegetables** in which there are **green leafy** vegetables (lettuce, endives, celery, etc.) which supply folic acid (necessary for the production of red cells in the blood), chlorophyll (rich in

A good breakfast with fresh fruits and dry cereals (or cooked breakfast foods), greatly favors physical and mental strength during the morning.

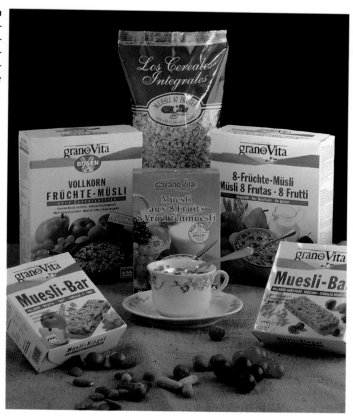

magnesium), minerals (especially iron) and trace elements.

The salad should also contain the **so-called colored** red and yellow vegetables, such as tomatoes, red peppers, beets and carrots, which supply **provitamin A** (carotenes) of great prophylactic value against cancer. Other vegetables such as onions, celery, radishes and raw cauliflower, as well as tender shoots of soybeans or alfalfa.

Vegetables used in a salad should be tender and cut into small pieces, to simplify the chewing process. They may be dressed with olive oil, preferably **olive** and **lemon** (rather than vinegar). Lovers of **vegetable condiments** may season their salad with marjoram, oregano, mint, etc.

Salt should be used *very **moderately,*** especially by those who suffer hypertension (no more than one teaspoon per day). Actually all vegetables contain enough mineral salts, including sodium chloride, so that there is no need of adding common salt to the salad. Furthermore, if it is dressed with lemon and/or herbs, salt will not be needed.

- An **energy-giving first course:** May be legumes (lentils, chickpeas, beans), pota-

Fresh fruit make up the ideal supper for an adult, especially if they wish to lose weight. Fruit combines very well with whole wheat toast, which makes it even more digestible.

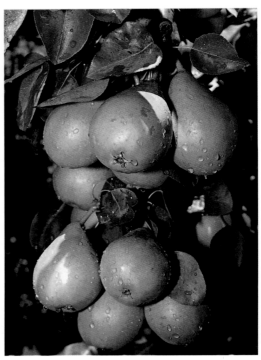

toes, grains (rice, oats, etc.) A legume and a cereal may be combined (for example, lentils with rice, or chickpeas with rice) in order to obtain a very high quality biological protein, similar to that of meat.

- A **second protein course** (vegetarian meat, products derived from soy meat, eggs) with other vegetables (peppers, artichokes, mushrooms, etc.)

- A **dessert** based on a piece or ration of fruit, such as an apple, pear, peach, strawberries, cherries, watermelon, etc.

Supper

This is **not always necessary** for all *adults,* because with a breakfast and a noon meal such as we have described, the nutritive needs of most persons are covered. Children and those who perform intense physical labor are exceptions to this general rule.

Abstaining from supper provides a longer rest period to the digestive system, and permits better assimilation of foods eaten during the day. Furthermore, not eating supper is the best way of losing weight. Generally calories which are ingested in the evening increase the body weight more than when taken in the morning.

In any case supper, if eaten, should be light, *at least* **2 hours** before retiring. The digestive processes are halted during sleep, so that if supper is eaten late, foods remain in the stomach. This creates digestive fermentation, which are manifested by a sour taste in the mouth, bad breath, or a heavy stomach. Furthermore, an individual sleeps better when the stomach does not have to perform a heavy duty.

For an adult, supper should be basically **fresh fruit.** A fruit salad with some crack-

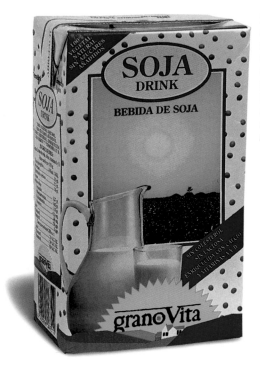

Soybean milk provides proteins of a high biological quality, as well as minerals and vitamins, and can therefore substitute cow milk, with the advantage that it does not contain cholesterol or saturated fats. The market place has soy milk enriched with calcium and vitamins A and D.

ers or whole wheat toast makes a good supper. Some may prefer to add yogurt or cottage cheese. Others prefer a more fatty dish of hot vegetable soup. And others choose a vegetable plate, such as asparagus, artichokes, or spinach smothered with young garlic, although is better to eat vegetables at the other meals of the day.

Whatever the case may be, it should be **light,** which really means containing **little fat.**

Children, young people who are in the developmental stage, persons who perform heavy physical work, and pregnant or breast-feeding women may need to eat a more substantial supper. To what has been mentioned, they may add products derived from soybeans, eggs, milk, yogurt, cottage cheese or nuts.

Begin the Day Properly

Breakfast should be the ***most important*** meal of the day for two basic reasons:

- **To replace reserves that have been used up** during the night. Although our body rests as we sleep, there are many organs and processes that do not cease working. These need energy: the heart, the lungs, and the body temperature are some of them. The body obtains energy for these processes beginning with the reserve of glycogen which is in the liver and is transformed into glucose during the night. Thus in the morning our energy reserves are lower and need to be replaced.

- It **provides** sufficient **energy** to work during the morning. Thus the sense of fainting or weakness will be avoided, so frequent at mid-morning, which many persons try to overcome mistakenly with a cup of coffee. This feeling of weakness is due to the lowering of the concentration of glucose in the blood. We normally have 0.8 to 1 gram of glucose per liter of blood (80 to 100 mg per 100 ml), and when this level goes down, the results are fatigue and a lower ability for concentration. Remember that the brain needs a continuous supply of glucose and oxygen in order to function well.

Therefore, what must be done to maintain a good level of glucose in the blood the entire morning?

Eating a good breakfast is the best way of doing this. Eating between meals, snacking, would be another way of maintaining the glucose level in the blood, but that is not a recommendable way: digestion is not carried on normally (the stomach needs a period of rest between two meals), digestive problems appear, appetite for food is reduced, and furthermore weight increases (generally the food taken in snacks is rich in sugar and fats).

We can fulfill these two objectives for eating breakfast by eating sweets: pastries, honey, fruits … And it works momentarily. But these simple sugars are metabolized swiftly, and within a very short time hunger appears again.

On the other hand, when **complex carbohydrates** (glucides) are eaten as found in cereals (especially whole grain) these are slowly transformed into glucose, and so the correct level in the blood is maintained for several hours.

Will a deficient breakfast affect our activities?

The first investigation that documented this was the famous *Iowa Study,* published in 1962. Children who went to school without breakfast revealed a lessening of their physical capacity (as measured by their consumption of oxygen), their endurance to effort, their muscular strength and their abili-

Painful Hunger

Some persons feel an irresistible hunger which even becomes painful, with an intense sensation of emptiness in the stomach eased only by eating. This generally happens at night, often after retiring.

This is a symptom of **gastroduodenal ulcer.** This is due to an excess of gastric juices in the stomach which irritate the lining, provoking violent contractions known as hunger pains. In this case, yes, we recommend eating supper. It would be good to eat a small quantity of cold alkalinizing foods, such as:

- Cold milk.
- Bananas or apples.
- Crackers or cereals.

Very hot foods, spices, coffee, fried and heavy foods should be avoided.

Nevertheless, wanting a solution to the problem, the sufferer should go to his doctor, who may diagnose a possible gastroduodenal ulcer and apply a treatment.

ty to concentrate and learn. It seems very clear that **children** should go to school after eating a breakfast which represents at least **20%** to **25%** of the total caloric value of the **daily diet,** and which is made up of varied foods, according to the groups of foods (see page 141).

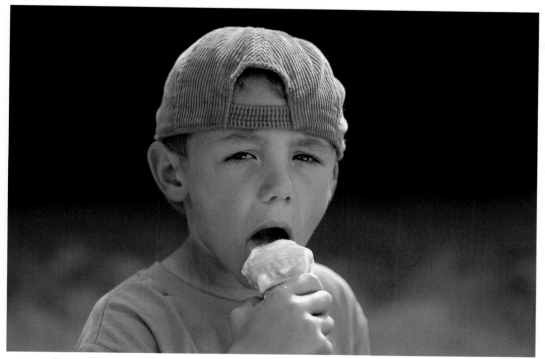

To be able to really enjoy food and good health, the appetite must be educated and subjected to the will. Thanks to this self-control of the appetite, which is based on temperance, we can resist snacking between meals, eating that which we know will do us harm, and overeating. Temperance is abstinence from everything harmful and moderate use of that which is healthful.

What if I have no appetite when I get up?

Undoubtedly you are not hungry in the morning if you ate a large supper, or ate it very late. Begin to cut down on your supper, and eating it earlier, and you will soon discover that you will wake up with an appetite. This change should be made gradually.

Soybeans, an Exceptional Legume

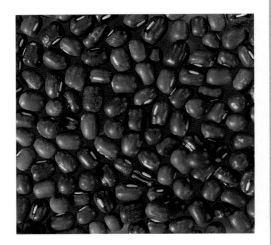

The soybean plant is a leguminous plant, which grows to around one metre high. There are varieties that have black, green or red beans. For over two thousand years, along with rice, it has formed the basic diet of the people of East and Southeast Asia where very little meat, milk and eggs are consumed. Thanks to the soybean plant, these oriental peoples have been able to cover all their nutritional requirements. The soybean plant is the **star of vegetable foods.** The following elements are found in its composition:

- A very important percentage of **high biological quality** of **proteins** (up to 40% of the dry weight of the bean), which contains **all** of the **essential amino acids.**

- A relatively important amount of **fats** (up to 20%), formed principally of **polyunsaturated fatty acids.** Among these is found the **linoleic acid,** an essential fatty acid which fulfills important functions in the body (see page 52).

- **Lecithin** (around 2%), an important phospholipid for the function of the **nervous system,** which also contributes to the lowering of the blood **cholesterol** level, as well as many other functions.

Soybean proteins can be compared to those of meat with regards to their nutritional value, to the point that they may even substitute meat. Even **nursing babies,** who need a supply of essential amino acids, may be raised satisfactorily with soybean milk enriched with vitamin B_{12} and calcium in case they are allergic to cow milk.

The soybean is a food of great nutritive value, which **should not be eaten excessively.** It need not be eaten daily, an error into which some fall when they shift to a vegetarian diet and are afraid they will not get enough proteins. Though we are dealing with a vegetable, we should not think that we are dealing with a product of little or "light" food value.

Products Derived From the Soybean

Product	Description	Use
Sprouts	The tender sprouts of soybean. They are found in stores and can also be made at home.	Can be used raw in salads and desserts. They are very rich in **vitamins, enzymes, chlorophyll,** as well as **proteins** with the advantage that when eaten **raw,** the maximum of all its nutritive properties are avalaible.
Flour	Composed of ground soybeans. It can be found in stores, with or without the soybean fat.	In pastries, pasta and desserts. When added to wheat flour, it enhances its nutritional value. It allows one to replace **eggs** in pastries, **with the advantage** of not having cholesterol.
Milk	Is made of soybeans which are ground, cooked, and filtered. In stores it is also known as soy drink.	Can **replace cow milk** with the **advantage** of not containing animal fats or cholesterol. It is rich in essential fatty acids, specially linoleic (see page 52). Its content of **iron, vitamin B₁** (thiamin) and **niacin** is higher than that of cow milk. On the other hand, soymilk contains less calcium than cow milk. In the market there are some soymilks enriched with this mineral and vitamins A and D.
Oil	High quality table oil with a neutral flavor. It has up to 61% polyunsaturated fatty acids (see page 145).	Flavors salads, pastries and cooking in general.
Tofu	It is **soy cheese.** It is prepared by adding a coagulant to soybean milk (for example: lemon), and applying pressure for several days until it acquires a semi-solid state.	It is used in the place of white cheese. It has a neutral taste, which makes it very useful in many cooked foods. It must be seasoned with salt and consistency.
Sauce (tamari)	Fermented soybeans, water and marine salt. The fermentation process requires 6 to 12 months.	It is used moderately as a condiment.
Meat substitude	It may contain soy grains or may be combined with cereal flour or nuts. There are many kinds and tastes: steaks, hamburgers, sausages, etc.	As a meat substitute, especially in transitional diets (see page 171). It has **all the advantages of meat** in protein content, but **without its inconveniences.**

Counsels on Cooking

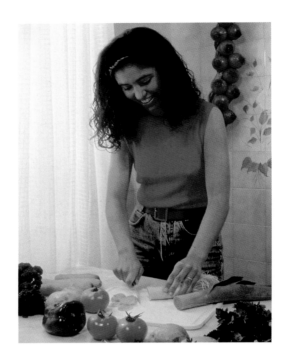

When You Go Shopping

- Choose **unrefined products,** such as bread, pasta, whole grains, as well as brown sugar and unrefined or iodized salt.
- Purchase foods that have a **low fat content,** such as milk, yogurt, and low-fat cheese.
- **Read the labels** on the items you purchase, especially noticing their content of fat, sugar, salt, and additives.

In Preparing Your Menus

- **Use egg white** instead of the whole egg (the yolk has abundant cholesterol) to make foods adhere together.
- **Use less and less butter,** and more vegetable oil.
- **Margarine** is preferable to butter. Since it is of plant origin, it has no cholesterol, although it contains saturated fatty acids (hydrogenated). **Vegetable oils** contain unsaturated fatty acids, which lower the level of blood cholesterol.
- **Reduce the amount of meat** in stews. Try substituting it with legumes or soybean derivatives.
- If you do eat meat, **eliminate all visible fats** that you can, and leave aside all the skin of fowls, which have a lot of fat.
- Take advantage of the **foods that are in season,** with the goal of eating **fresh products** as much as possible.
- Aim at having **a contrast in colors and taste** in presenting the food. This stimulates the digestive juices and favors digestion.
- **Avoid repeating** of the same food in the same meal, for example, eggs and custard, or noodle soup and macaroni.

How to Cook vegetables

- **Eat raw** vegetables as much as possible. In this way their food value, mineral salts, vitamins and enzymes are best utilized. Of course this requires good teeth as well as careful chewing. You will discover new and refreshing flavors. Have you tried raw and tender artichoke hearts, cut in pieces and dressed with oil and lemon? Or raw mushrooms in the salad? And grated carrots, well dressed?

- **Avoid fried foods:** Overheated or re-used oil is usually converted into various irritating chemical substances, especially acrolein, which leads to slow and heavy digestion. If you must fry, use **olive oil,** which is more stable at high temperatures, and takes longer to oxidize and decompose than seed oils.

- Vegetables **baked in an oven** (wood, electric, or gas) are very tasty and digestible. Try baking red peppers, eggplant, leeks, onions and potatoes. Prepare them with drops of oil and a bit of sliced garlic.

- **Steaming** or microweving foods are also good ways of cooking vegetables, although they may not be as tasty as those prepared in conventional ovens. The **microwave** has been accused of producing chemical changes in food. Although it has not been proven convincingly, it is well to be prudent in the use of this appliance.

- When you cook vegetables, do it with **the least quantity of water possible,** for water dilutes the vitamins and mineral salts. At any rate, use **the broth of the vegetables** as a soup, or to take it as a hot drink in wintertime.

To Avoid the Destruction of Vitamins by Cooking

- **Let the water boil** before tossing in the vegetables. Thus the oxygen which is generally found throughout the water is freed, and does not oxidize the vitamins in the foods. Oxidation presupposes the loss of vitamins.

- **Do not peel the skin** of vegetables (such as potatoes, turnips, or carrots), for these keep vitamins from leaving the food to be dissolved in the water.

- **Cut the vegetables in small pieces.** This will simplify their cooking. Larger pieces require more time for cooking, resulting in a greater destruction of the vitamins by heat.

- Try to **eat** cooked vegetables **as soon as possible.** What is left should be kept in the refrigerator, protected from contact with the air in a closed receptacle or wrapped in a sheet of plastic or aluminum paper. The oxygen in the air provokes the destruction of vitamins through oxidation.

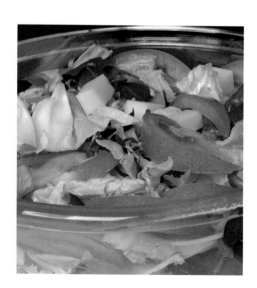

The Mediterranean Diet

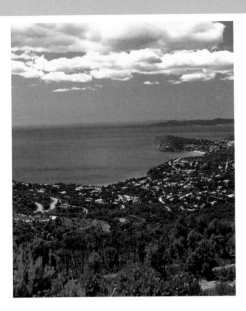

The traditional diet of the regions bordering the Mediterranean, rich in vegetables, legumes and fish, has been demonstrated as being more healthful than the countries in central and northern Europe, where meat and milk products are eaten in abundance.

Traditionally, in areas of the Mediterranean, especially in those near the coast, another kind of diet is followed that is different from that of central and northern Europe and in the United States. These dietary habits typical of the southern part of the old continent, known as the "Mediterranean diet," are still in vogue because they have demonstrated that they protect from cardiovascular diseases and against certain kinds of cancer.

The typical Mediterranean diet is still followed in the rural areas and the coasts of southern Europe. Unfortunately, some of these good dietary habits are disappearing in the urban and industrial areas. Nevertheless, as the advantages of the traditional Mediterranean diet have been discovered, interest has increased, and many wish to return to the ancestral customs of the inhabitants of "Mare Nostrum."

The Mediterranean diet has the following characteristics:

- **An abundant use of grains, fruits, legumes and vegetables.** A fresh vegetable salad is an ever-present item in the noon meal.
- **Use of olive oil,** instead of butter, lard, or other animal fats, to dress all kinds of foods.
- **Moderate use of animal products,** preferring fish over meat, and limiting the use of milk and its derivatives.

The consumption of fruits and vegetables per person in the Mediterranean regions is double that of the countries of central and northern Europe; on the other hand the use of meat and milk is much less. Up to a few years ago it was thought the Anglo-Saxon diet was the ideal one, with an abundance of proteins and animal products, which favor the rapid growth of children, and a good appearance in the youth: The tall northern blondes were admired by the people of southern Europe.

Nevertheless, when it became known that this typical diet of the inhabitants of central and northern Europe was responsible, among other things, for the great number of cardiac and degenerative problems that exist in those countries, investigators have fixed their attention on the apparently poorer diet that is traditionally followed in the Mediterranean areas.

The Mediterranean diet contains **less fats, less proteins,** and **more carbohydrates** than the typical western diet, as is now recommended by the WHO. Furthermore, **unsaturated acid fats,** which are found in vegetable oils and in fish, predominate over the saturated fatty acids which are found in meat and milk products.

The so-called Mediterranean diet is much more healthful than the typical meat diet of industrialized countries. Nevertheless, the **results** obtained with this diet are **surpassed** by the **diet based entirely on vegetables,** as stated elsewhere in this book. The **greater** the **proportion** of **grains, fruits** and **plant foods** (including legumes and vegetables) in the diet, the **more healthful it will be.**

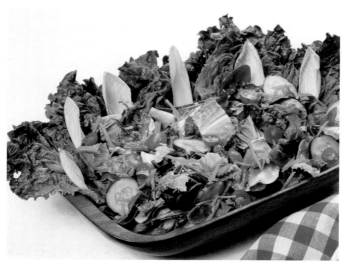

A fresh raw vegetable salad, dressed with olive oil, is a basic element of the Mediterranean diet.

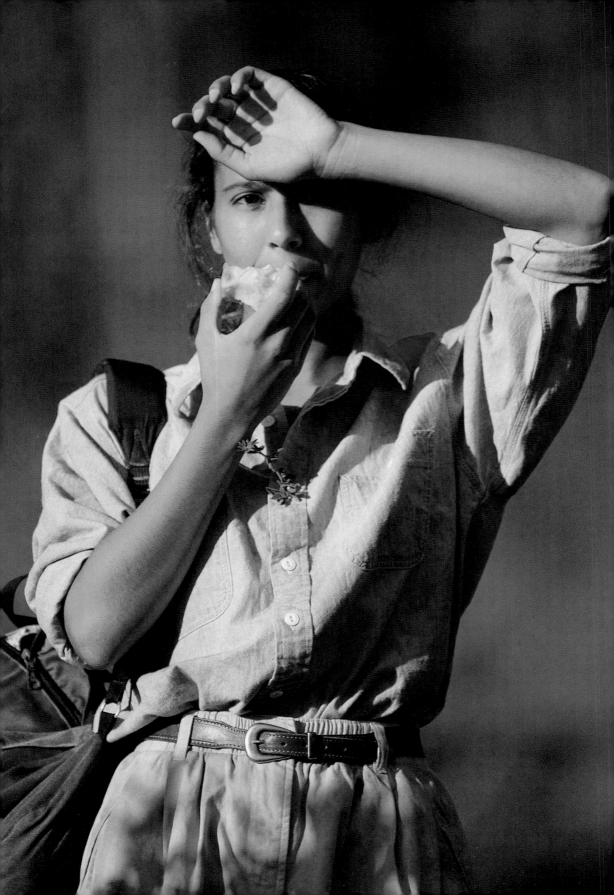

14

Those Who Lose, Win

EXPERIENCE tells us, and statistics confirm, that rarely will we find an obese vegetarian. In fact, obesity or the tendency toward it is one of the good reasons to change diet and base it on plant foods.

Excess weight creates many health problems. The heart, the bones and the joints are overloaded in their functions. To lose weight is to gain health. It has been said that one kilo more of weight represents one year less of life.

Obesity is the result of an imbalance between energy that is ingested and that which the body really needs. The energy that is left over accumulates in the form of fats, especially under the skin.

Seen in this way, there are only two solutions to avoid excess weight: take in less calories and use more calories. Nevertheless this is not as simple as it seems, and there are other factors which decisively affect the problem of overweight.

continues on page 161

> **In the control of appetite, we should think of the average. If the body is very fat, the weight is hard to carry, and if it is too thin, it cannot carry us.**
>
> **ST. FRANCIS OF SALES**
> Bishop of Geneva
> 1567-1622

Consumption of Calories per Hour
in Different Physical Activities

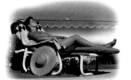

Sleep: 65

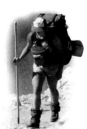

Walking: 250

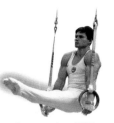

Gymnastics: 350

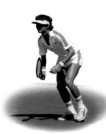

Tennis: 450

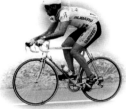

Cycling: 500

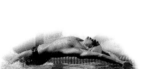

Swimming: 650

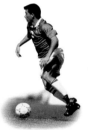

Soccer: 850

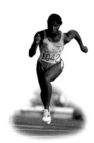

Racing: 1.000

Daily Need of Calories According to the Activity

Type of Activity	Professions	Calories Consumed Daily
Sedentary or very light	Office workers, teachers	1,800
Light	Students, salesmen, domestic labor (with electric appliances)	2,300
Moderate	Mechanics, carpenters domestic labor (without elesctric appliances)	2,800
Intense	Construction workers, miners, athletes	3,500 +

That Which is More Fatterning

- **Fats,** especially those of animal origin.

- **Refined carbohydrates,** such as white flour and sugar, as well as products containing these items: Pastries, rolls, confections.

- **Alcoholic beverages,** especially beer. Alcohol contains abundant calories which are transformed into fat.

- **Excess salt in the diet.** Salt retains water, and this increases weight.

continues from page 159

Causes of Obesity
Not All the Causes Are Listed

"I do not understand why I am getting fat, with the little that I eat!"

Have you not heard this said at some time? Very often fat people are accused of eating too much. But actually this is not the only nor most important cause of obesity. All of us have known thin persons who eat abundantly. There are even those who try to gain weight, but fail.

There must be, therefore, aside from eating too much food, other factors which cause obesity. There is a classic experiment which investigators of human nutrition know well: Eating exactly the same, and carrying on the same daily exercise program, some persons increase in weight, others maintain weight, and others may even become thinner. Not all persons gain weight at the same rate. The causes of these differences between individuals are as yet not clear, in spite of the great amount of research done on this subject. But the following are indicated:

- There is a **hereditary factor.** There are individuals who have inherited from their ancestors a corpulent constitution, which may possibly be related to a better assimilation of food. A child of fat parents has an 80% chance of also being fat, because they probably also will eat like their parents.

- There are **individual factors** which depend on the **hormonal balance** of each person. Hormones such as thyroxine, produced by the thyroid gland, speeds the combustion of nutrients in the body. On the contrary, insulin, increases the lipogenesis (production of fats). It has been proven that the obese are less sensitive to insulin, that is, they need more insulin to metabolize glucose. As a result, this causes an increase in the production of fat.

- The obese have a **smaller thermogenic capacity,** that is, they produce less heat than thin people.[1] The calories that are not transformed into energy accumulate in the body in the form of fat. To the contrary, thin persons spend more calories in trying to keep the body warm so they consume more energy and have a smaller deposit of fat.

- It would appear that individuals who tend to be obese have a **more sensitive hunger center,** a nerve nucleus which regulates the appetite and which is found in the hypothalamus, in the center of the brain. This makes them get hungry more often, and need more food to enjoy the feeling of fullness.

---

1. GRANDE COVIÁN, F. *Nutrición y salud* (Nutrition and Health). Madrid, Ediciones Temas de Hoy, 1990, page 47.

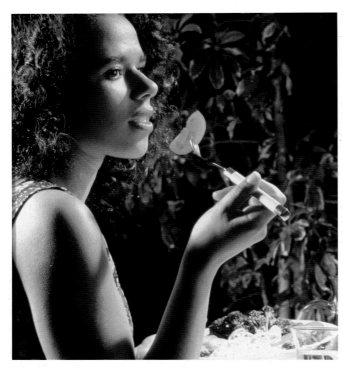

Salads are liable to be prepared in different ways and to be presented attractively. They provide a very important amount of vitamins and minerals with scarce calories. Because of this, they should be part of the daily menu in the weight reduction diets.

Weight Reduction Diets

At any rate, food plays a very important role whether the obesity is produced simply by overeating, or whether it is a result of individual predisposition. Nevertheless it is necessary to restrict the total amount of food, eliminate foods which have more fats and calories, and, in effect, reeducate dietary habits.

So that a weight loss diet may be effective and tolerated by the body, it should *fulfill* four basic objectives:

1. Reduce the total number of calories that are ingested, that is, reduce the total amount of food. It must be remembered that the body needs a minimum amount of energy to perform its basic functions, even though no exercise is involved. Using the automobile as a comparison, this minimum energy corresponds to the fuel that the idling motor of a stopped car uses.

The human body needs around **70 calories** per **hour** to cover the basic needs to maintain life, which is known as **basal metabolism.** Thus when asleep, 65 calories are spent per hour. If we remained in bed the entire day of 24 hours, without doing anything, we would need 65 x 24 = **1,560 calories per day** just to **maintain life.**

The sedentary life of an office worker who walks only when it is necessary, for example, does not require more than 2,000 calories per day. Any calories over this number that are ingested are transformed into fats which are stored away. For example, if a person needs 2,000 calories per day and ingests 2,900, he accumulates an excess of 900 calories which are equivalent to 100 grams of fat. If on the contrary he consumes less calories than necessary for basal metabolism, the body is forced to use up its own reserves.

continues on page 164

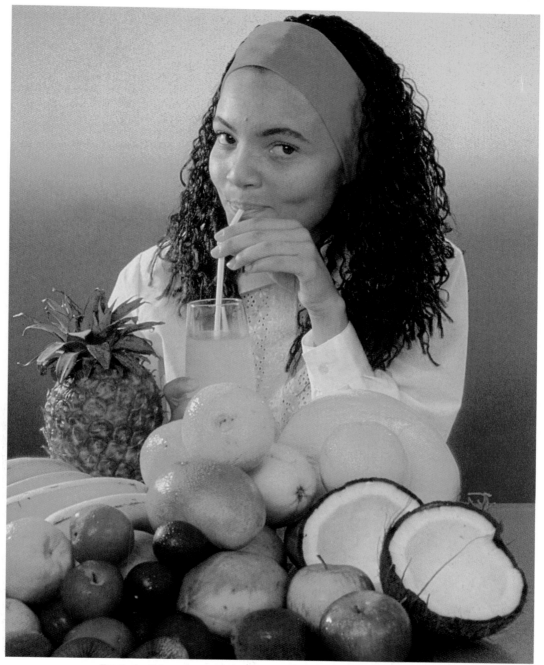

Fresh fruit is a necessary component of a weight-loss diet, for they contain vitamins and minerals and prevent constipation.

continues from page 162

The total of calories which a person needs each day, *never less* than 1,560, varies depending on several factors: the body weight (the heavier the person is, the more calories he will need), the sex (women need 10% less energy than men), and, above all, it depends upon the kind of exercise performed. The exact calculation of these quantities requires the knowledge of a specialist in nutrition.

2. Maintain an adequate proportion among the different caloric nutrients tending toward reducing the fat to the minimum that is recommended (see page 48).

Our bodies cannot feed only upon carbohydrates, or only upon fats and proteins. Theoretically this might be possible, since each one of these nutrients can provide the needed calories. But if this were done, this would result in metabolic unbalance. We must eat a variety of foods, and, furthermore, calories coming from each one of these nutrients must maintain a certain proportion: **carbohydrates,** from **55%** to **75%; fats,** from **15%** to **30%;** and **proteins,** from **10%** to **15%** (see page 34).

This implies **weight loss diets** such as the **Atkins** program, which consists of the total elimination of all carbohydrates and unlimited consumption of fats and proteins, are not recommended. With such a diet, a loss of a few kilos may be noticed, especially during the first few days; but this is due to the fact that there is a greater loss of water and calories through the urine.[2] These calories are lost in the form of proteins and ketonic bodies (acetone) which are eliminated through the urine in high quantities. Furthermore a diet rich in fats and proteins causes constipation, increases cholesterol, acidifies the blood, and causes a great upset of the metabolism in the organism, from which many cannot recover.

There are other unbalanced diets which claim to lead to weight loss that are equally harmful to health, which also alter the ideal proportion between caloric nutrients: carbohydrates, fats and proteins. For example, the **disassociated diet** or the separation diet, in which carbohydrates and proteins may not be eaten together; and the **macrobiotic** diet on its higher level, in which only cereals may be eaten.

3. Reduce to the recommended minimum (15%) the proportion of calories from fats, *eliminating* those from animal origin. These are saturated fats, solid at room temperature (such as bacon), which tend to be deposited in the consumer, in the same place where they were found in the animal from which they came: just under the skin, in what is called the subcutaneous cellular tissue.

On the contrary, plant fats or **oils** become liquid at room temperature, and our organism metabolizes them with greater facility than that of animals. This means that vegetable oils are transformed more easily into energy and do not have as marked a character as a reserve food (see page 46).

Plant foods based on soybeans have many advantages over meat, not only in the weight-loss diets, but in general for all people. Soy contains complete proteins with all of the essential amino acids, and further it has no cholesterol. Because it has less fat, calories from soy products are proportionately inferior to those of meat and its derivatives (see table on page 166). We are dealing with healthful foods that are pleasant to the taste, which provide nutrients at a proportion satisfactory for a weight-loss program.

It is recommended that the **substitution** of meat products by plant foods be done *progressively* so that the organism and the palate may adapt to a new type of food.

---

2. GRANDE COVIÁN, F. *Ibid*, page 59.

4. Increase breakfast, and cut down or even eliminate supper. Calories which are assimilated in the morning will be consumed easily throughout the day. This does not happen with those which are eaten at night, if after having supper one retires. You will find on page 143 the way of starting the day with a good breakfast.

Lose Weight, but Safely

With a diet based on vegetables, the five requirements for an efficient and safe diet can easily be reached from the health standpoint:

1. **Plant foods are generally less concentrated** than those of animal origin, so with an equal weight, they contain less calories. This makes it more difficult to take in excess calories when dealing with a vegetarian diet, since it would be necessary to fill the stomach excessively.

2. **A varied vegetarian diet provides all necessary nutrients in an adequate proportion** to lose weight, according to the chart found on page 34. An excessive amount of proteins and fats are consumed in a **meat diet,** at the same time reducing the proportion of carbohydrates. This causes a greater elimination of calcium through the urine (see pages 85, 121). The rich protein diet may damage the kidneys.

3. **Complex carbohydrates** such as those found in whole cereals, used in adequate quantities and proportion, do not cause obesity, as many think, but are ***indispensable*** in a balanced weight loss program. Simple carbohydrates such as sugars are not good, especially when accompanying fats, as often happens in pastries and candies.

4. **Vegetable foods generally have less fats than animal foods.** This permits that the total fats in the diet be less, which is a requirement for weight loss.

5. **Fats in vegetable foods are generally of the unsaturated type and are beneficial** to health, contrary to that of animal fats. Fats should not be totally eliminated from the diet, for they contain essential fatty acids which fulfill functions that cannot be substituted in the body (see page 52), found above all in vegetable oils.

Comparative Chart of Vegetable Products Based on Soybeans and Those Based on Meat

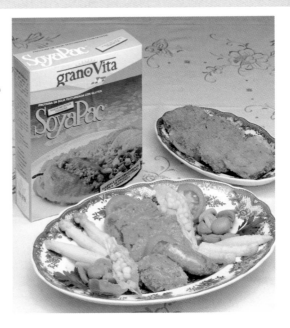

Food	Carbohydrates	fats	proteins	Cholesterol	Calories
Protein vegetable steaks	4,84	0,14	20,42	0	102
Beef-steak	0	10,5	19,2	85	177
Vegeburger	7,1	4,6	25	0	165
Hamburger (meat)	0	14,0	22,5	70	216
Soy meats	3,8	6,1	12,4	0	120
Lean pork ribs	0	18,1	26,1	96	271
Texturized protein foods	29,9	0,5	50,6	0	323
Cooked york ham	0,3	39,6	16,2	85	435
Vegetarian wieners	4	16	11	0	204
Frankfurt sausages	2	20	14	100	248

The figures refer to grams for each 100 grams of food. Cholesterol is given in mg per 100 grams. The last column in calorie units.

Carbohydrates

Vegetarian products based on soybeans	Though they are **fundamentally protein foods,** they **contain some** of **carbohydrates.** This draws them nearer to the ideal proportion which should exist between the caloric nutrients (carbohydrates, fats and proteins) as shown in the chart on page 34. Carbohydrates are necessary in all diets including weight loss diets. In their absence the body has to burn up fats and proteins, which results in ketonic bodies and other residual acids which alter the metabolism.
Meat and its derivatives	**Do not** contain **carbohydrates,** or only in a very small quantity (the viscera such as the liver). This makes a regimen based on meat unbalanced in the proportion of needed nutrients.

Fats

Vegetarian products based on soybeans	Contain much **less fat** than meat, and furthermore the fat is of a **higher** nutritive **quality,** and **fattens less.**
Meat and its derivatives	Have a **large amount of saturated fats,** harmful to health (see page 46) and favor the **increase of weight.**

Proteins

Vegetarian products based on soybeans	The **proportion** of proteins is **similar** to or even superior to that of meat. Furthermore, the proteins in soy are **complete.**
Meat and its derivatives	Are a good source of **complete proteins.**

Cholesterol

Vegetarian products based on soybeans	**No vegetable food** contains cholesterol.
Meat and its derivatives	They are **rich in cholesterol.** It is recommended that no more than **300 mg per day** of cholesterol be ingested, a quantity that is easily reached and surpassed in meat foods.

Calories

Vegetarian products based on soybeans	At the same weight and quantity of proteins, vegetable foods provide **less calories.** This makes them especially suited to **weight-loss** diets.
Meat and its derivatives	The caloric content is **high** due to higher percentage of **fat.**

Avoid Constipation

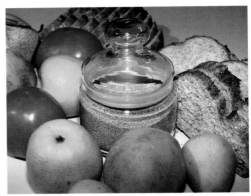

Constipation often follows a typical weight-loss program, especially when it includes a large amount of meat, fish and milk with its derivatives, none of which contain cellulose or vegetable fiber (see page 43), substances indispensable to the good performance of the intestines. Fruit and whole cereals are the best source of fiber.

Most of the cases of constipation are of functional origin, either a weakness in the intestinal muscles or an inadequate diet. Nevertheless do not forget that when constipation appears suddenly, it may be a symptom of a serious intestinal disease, for example, colon cancer.

Chronic constipation should be corrected by dietetic-hygiene measures. The intestines should be reeducated, and their muscles should be strengthened in order to favor the progression of the feces. Here are some counsels to overcome constipation:

- Drink one or two glasses of **water** on getting up. Continue drinking water during the rest of the day, at least four to six additional glasses.
- Eat a **breakfast with whole cereals and bread,** fresh fruit, fruit jam and several **dried prunes.** The latter can be soaked during the night and eaten, together with the water in which they were soaked.
- Eat **fresh fruit** in abundance during the day, especially grapes, apples, cherries, strawberries and peaches.
- In persistent cases take one or two spoonfuls of **bran** in the morning. Bran is a type of vegetable fiber which is found in cereals (see page 41). Do not go beyond two spoonfuls per day, neither take it over long periods of time, since bran makes the absorption of iron and other minerals difficult in the intestines. If cereals and whole wheat breads are eaten, these already have a balanced portion of bran.
- **Avoid astringent foods** such as non-whole crackers, white bread, pasta, eggs, and such drinks as wine or tea.
- Carry on a regular **physical exercise** program. The one which gives the best results is a fast walk a half hour each day.
- Get your body accustomed to evacuate at a **fixed hour** each day.

Examples of Weight-loss Menus

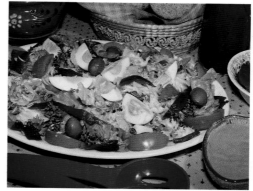

For weight-loss programs to be healthful, they should maintain an ideal proportion among the different energy-providing nutrients (carbohydrates, fats and proteins). This implies that they should be varied, not restricted to only a few kinds of foods.

1,000 Calorie Daily Diet

Breakfast

Soy milk or skimmed milk . . . . .1 glass
Wheat germ or pollen . . . . .1 tablespoonful
Cereales integrales (muesli) . . . . . . .2 tablespoonful
Walnuts or almonds . . . . .30 grams
Oranges 1
Other fresh fruits 1

Noon Meal

Mixed vegetable salad
Olive or vegetable seed oil . . . . .1 tablespoonful
Vegetarian meat
    with vegetables . . . . .200 grams
Dextrinized whole wheat . . . . .2 slices
Baked apple 1

Supper

Fruit salad
    (without sugar or honey) . . . . .1 ration
Whole crackers . . . . .100 grams
Brewer's yeast . . . . .1 tablespoonful

1,500 Calorie Daily Diet

Breakfast

Fruit juice . . . . .1 glass
Cereal with
    dried fruit . . . . .3 tablespoonful
Tofu (soy cheese), cottage cheese or yogurt
Wheat germ or pollen . . . . .1 tablespoonful
Whole bread with a low
    calorie jam . . . . .1 slice

Noon Meal

Mixed vegetable salad
Olive or vegetable seeds oil . . . . .1 tablespoonful
A bowl of vegetable soup
    or a portion of legumes
Vegetarian sausages 2
    or one boiled egg
Dextrinized whole wheat bread . . . . .2 slices
Seasonal fruit 1

Supper

Vegetable soup with onion and celery . . . . . .1 plate
Nuts or dried fruit . . . . .30 grams
Seasonal fruit 2

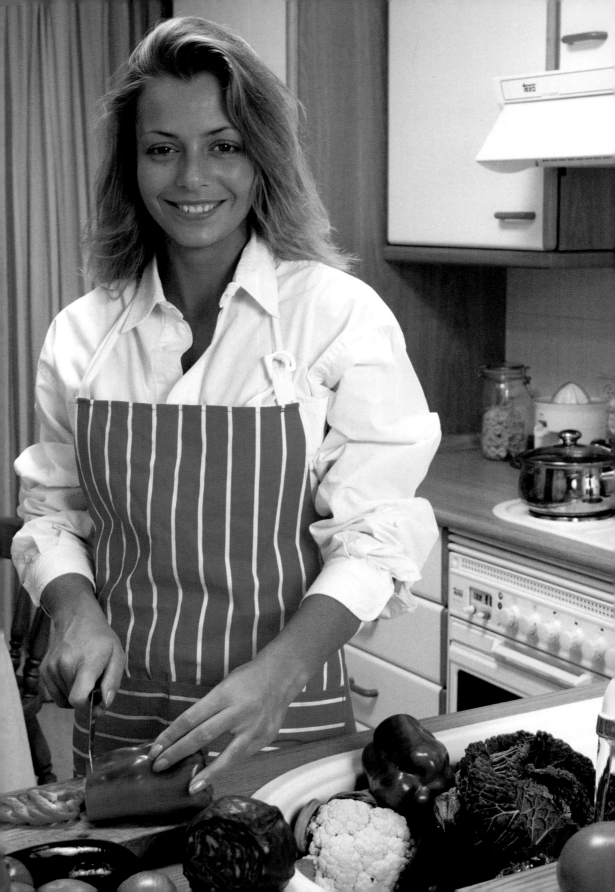

15

The Transition Diet

AFTER EXAMINING all that has been written up to this point, many of the readers may ask: *What must I do to eat better? How may I substitute meat and its derivatives, which I may be eating in excess?*

In the first place we should say that a meat diet cannot be blamed for all diseases. But it is a very important risk factor, as has been demonstrated, in some of them (cardiocirculatory diseases and cancer, above all). But the vegetarian diet is not a panacea that is going to free us from all evils. It only helps us to be more healthy within the logical limitations of each individual. Further, perhaps it may increase your sensitivity toward yourself, and toward animals and nature in general.

If for any of the motives of health, ethics or ecology that have been explained (see page 115) you decide to change your dietary habits to a diet based on fruits, cereals and

**If you are planning for one year, plant rice.
If you are doing it for ten years, plant trees.
If you are doing it for a lifetime, educate a person.**

CHINESE PROVERB

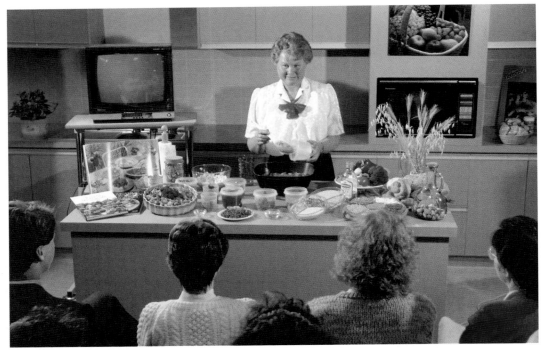

The attendance at a vegetarian cooking class is a good way to facilitate the change to a new style of healthful living.

vegetables, take into consideration the following counsels:

- **Convince yourself** that a vegetarian diet, especially if it is complemented with non-fat milk products and an occasional egg, provides all the elements necessary for proper nutrition. Forget the beliefs and prejudices of previous times when it was thought that meat was indispensable, or that those who ate vegetables were anemic and undernourished. To do so you will have to read and become sufficiently informed.

- **Attend a vegetarian cooking school** among those offered by different organizations. In this way you will discover tasty and healthful foods which may be prepared without recurring to meat products.

- **Introduce changes gradually.** Your body will take some time to become accustomed and adapt to the new foods. Your palate too.

If you discard meat suddenly, you will notice a sensation of weakness, even though you take the needed proteins and other nutrients. This sensation is produced because meat contains puric bases, with a chemical composition and effects similar to those of caffeine which produces an artificial stimulus. There are those who have come to compare meat with a drug, because it creates habit and dependency, and when its intake is halted, it provokes an abstinence syndrome. So meat should be substituted little by little by other foods, thus allowing our bodies to become adapted.

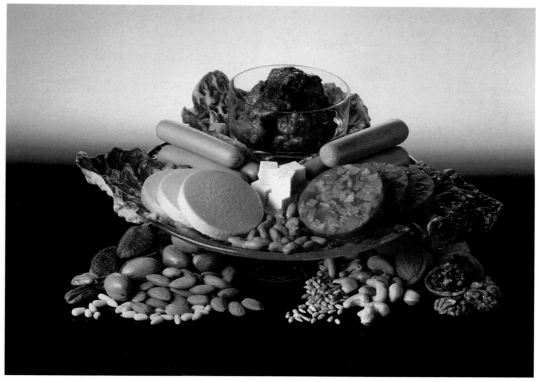

Vegetable products based on soybeans are a good substitute for meat. Nuts and gluten (wheat protein) are also good substitutes. They are especially helpful in transition diets, which endeavor to replace meat by more healthful plant products.

- **Try not to eat too much.** Meat foods produce a feeling of fullness in the stomach due to the fact that its digestion is slower.

  When you begin to eat cereals, fruits and other plant foods, you may have the sensation of not having had enough to eat, although actually this is not so. This will last for only a short time, and very soon your digestive system will learn how to be satisfied with healthier foods.

- **Try to season your foods** using healthful vegetable condiments such as oregano, sage or cumin. Saturated fats of animal origin (the most unhealthful) enhance the taste of the foods and excite the taste buds. At the beginning, when you omit these, it may be that you will feel a lack of taste in the foods, but the vegetable condiments will make the change easier.

- **Begin by omitting the stronger meats,** that is, those which have a greater fat content and those which overload the organism. These are:

  ✓ **Pork,** which without doubt is the most harmful for human consumption. This was already known by such ancient cultures as the Jewish and Moslem. Today we know that pork and its derivatives (sausages) are very rich in saturated animal fats, as well as cholesterol. Furthermore, because of the unsanitary conditions in which they are generally raised, hogs are frequently attacked by various diseases, from the porcine disease produced by a virus similar to that of the flu, to various parasitisms: trichina, cysticercosis, tapeworm, etc. Pork should be the first meat eliminated from your table.

✓ **Game meat,** especially the rabbit, even though it may come from a farm. They are strong meats, rich in uric acid and are hard to digest.

✓ **Shellfish,** in general, have much cholesterol, produce uric acid, and are indigestible. Furthermore, they often contain bacterial toxins, with which they are frequently contaminated.

Enjoy the Change

As the diet is changing toward a diet based on plant products, the body undergoes a series of processes of physiological adaptation. Sensations that are felt are varied, depending on the constitution of each individual. The following are some of the most frequent:

- *"I feel that I am digesting food better."*
- *"I notice that I am more agile and active."*
- *"For the first time I am losing weight without having to follow a strict diet."*
- *"I notice that I have less heartburn."*
- *"I have a daily bowel movement and do not need laxatives."*
- *"The nervousness and feeling of unrest which I used to have have disappeared."*

These and other health aspects are strengthened and enriched, when, aside from changing diet habits, seven other decisive factors are taken into consideration, listed in the first chapter of this book (page 13):

Order To Be Followed in Substituting Animal with Plant Foods

1 Change from **pork, rabbit,** or **shellfish to red meats** (lamb and beef) or white meats (chicken, duck, etc.).
↓
2 Change from red or white **meats to fish.**
↓
3 Change from **fish to milk, eggs** and **soy products.**
↓
4 Base your diet on **fruits, cereals,** and **plant foods** (which include vegetables, tubers and legumes) to enjoy better health.

- Breathing pure **air.**
- The use of plenty of **water** both inside and out.
- Adequate exposure to **sunlight.**
- Regular performance of physical **exercise.**
- Healing **rest,** daily, weekly, and annually.
- **Abstinence** from **toxins** (tobacco, alcohol, drugs).
- **Good mental attitude.**

174

Family Involvement

The **change** towards a vegetarian diet should be done **gradually,** and with the participation of the whole family.

As the body becomes adjusted to the vegetarian diet and new foods and culinary possibilities are discovered, derivatives of soybeans become less necessary, though they will always be a healthful and nutritive complement. The ideal is to eat vegetarian foods in their most natural state.

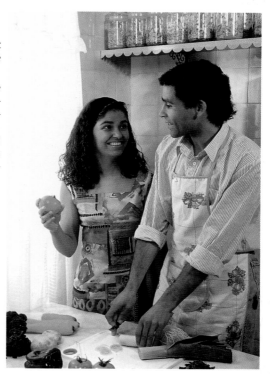

"Data generally indicates that a vegetarian diet carries with it less risk of chronic diseases than the present diets of prosperous communities."*

* WHO, Technical Report Series, No. 797, (*Diet, Nutrition, and the Prevention of Chronic Diseases*). Report of a WHO Study Group. Geneva, World Health Organization, 1990, page 109.

Obtain Maximum Benefit

Each human being enters the world with a *"health capital."* Some have more, some less. But each one should administer wisely those resources which nature has given him.

The **eight points** which we propose including a healthful diet, form an excellent program for life, and will allow us to obtain the maximum benefit of our initial *"health capital."* It is not an exaggeration to say that the larger part of diseases are directly related to our lifestyle. Remember that medicine and doctors will not be able to do for your health what you can do for yourself .

Dear reader: There are good reasons for following a **new lifestyle** which will include, among other things, a vegetarian diet. The positive results of such changes are recognized world-wide. The practical way of carrying these into effect, you already know.

A change to a more healthful lifestyle is possible. You may **enjoy** this change even now; it only depends on you.

TEST

Confirm Your Nutricional Knowledge

6. In order to lose weight it is necessary to follow a diet with many proteins and few carbohydrates.
   a. True.
   b. False.
   c. It depends on the metabolism of each person.

1. Vegetable fiber is:
   a. An important source of proteins.
   b. A useless waste that the intestines cannot absorb.
   c. A protective factor against colon cancer.

7. The iron which is found in legumes, vegetables and fruits:
   a. Is absorbed better than that proceeding from meat.
   b. May be sufficient to cover daily needs.
   c. Produces intolerance in the stomach.

2. Which one of these three foods has more protein content per 100 grams?
   a. Beef.
   b. Dry soybeans.
   c. Eggs.

8. Ham:
   a. Is a good source of polyunsaturated fatty acids.
   b. Is one of the more digestible meats.
   c. Contains nitrites and nitrates with a positive carcinogenic effect, but necessary for the preservation of ham.

3. Excess cholesterol in the blood may be due to a diet:
   a. Rich in olive oil.
   b. Abundant in butter and sausages.
   c. Rich in proteins.

9. Vegetarian athletes:
   a. Need animal protein supplements to be able to compete.
   b. Have greater resistance to fatigue than those who eat meat.
   c. Are able to develop greater strength at the starting time.

4. Meat is indispensable in a balanced and complete diet:
   a. Always.
   b. Never.
   c. Only for children.

5. The basic needs for vitamin C may be supplied using each day:
   a. One half kilo of meat.
   b. One liter of milk.
   c. One orange.

10. Osteoporosis (fragility of the bones):
    a. Is more frequent among vegetarian women.
    b. May be aggravated by a heavy intake of proteins.
    c. Is the result of a lack of iodine.

Answers to the Test

1:c. Vegetable fiber, which is made of cellulose, is not absorbed by the intestines, and for this reason, it was thought to be useless. But there is actually nothing really useless in natural foods. Each one of their components has its own function. The human intestines need residuals which cannot be assimilated in order to be able to function correctly, and their lack is the cause of numerous problems, among them colon cancer, constipation and intestinal diverticula (see page 43).

2:b. One hundred grams of dried soy beans contain 37 grams of protein of high biological value, comparable to meat proteins. 100 grams of meat provide from 15 to 21 grams of proteins, depending on the kind of meat. 100 grams of eggs have 13 grams of protein, that is, about 6 grams for each egg (see page 56).

3:b. Both butter and sausages are products especially rich in saturated fats and cholesterol. Olive oil, because it is a vegetable product, contains no cholesterol. The quantity of protein in the diet bears no relationship to the level of blood cholesterol.

Butter has 219 mg of cholesterol for each 100 grams, and sausages around 70. It is recommended that we should not consume over 300 mg per day of cholesterol (see pages 48, 49).

4:b. Neither adults, of whatever age, nor children need to eat meat in order to maintain a balanced and complete diet. Meat provides proteins of high biological value; but the proteins of cereals, nuts, legumes and vegetables, adequately combined among themselves have together the quantity and the proportion of necessary amino acids. Those who are not sure of their knowledge of adequately combining vegetable proteins, especially for children, need only to add milk and/or eggs to the vegetarian diet. Thus vegetable proteins are enriched, and the resulting diet is satisfactory (see page 63, 116).

As to vitamin B12 and iron, see pages 71 and 87 respectively.

5:c. An average-sized orange (200 grams) has 106 mg of vitamin C. According to the WHO, 60 mg are enough to cover daily needs. One liter of milk only contains 9.4 mg of vitamin C (0.94 mg per 100 ml), insufficient for the daily allowance. Meat, like eggs, does not contain vitamin C (see page 74).

6:b. This erroneous idea is the reason some endeavor to lose weight by eating fried beefsteak with vegetables. In order for a program of weight loss to be effective and not harmful to health, a correct proportion must be maintained among the different nutrients (see page 164), though it should be hypocaloric, that is, with a smaller quantity of each one of them.

7:b. Legumes, vegetables and fruits contain an abundant quantity of iron, sufficient to cover the daily needs of any individual. Nevertheless the absorption of iron from vegetables is more difficult than that from meat. However, this is compensated with the larger quantity of iron found in vegetables, and with the action of vitamin C which favors the absorption of iron (see page 88).

8:c. Ham and sausages are treated with nitrites and nitrates to avoid their putrefaction and to give them a more appetizing color. These additives may be converted into nitrosamines, known for its carcinogenic effect in the intestines (see page 137).

Ham contains above all saturated fats, not polyunsaturated. The latter are found in seed oils. Furthermore, pork generally has much collagen, the same as shellfish, which slows down digestion, causes intestinal putrefaction, and overloads the digestive system.

9:b. Athletes who eat vegetables rich in complex carbohydrates like whole cereals have a greater resistance to fatigue than those who eat proteins and fats of animal origin (see page 120), although their strength at a given moment may be less.

It has been demonstrated that physical exercise does not increase the need for proteins, unless there is a desire to abnormally develop the muscular volume (see page 60).

10:b. The ingestion of a high amount of proteins, as found in meat diets, increases the elimination of calcium through the urine, and may favor the development of osteoporosis (see page 85). Statistical studies reveal that osteoporosis is less frequent among vegetarian women.

Iodine has an effect upon the thyroid gland and upon the metabolism in general, but has no relationship to osteoporosis.

GLOSSARY

See also the Index

albumin/albuminoid: Terms which have been used traditionally as synonyms for "protein". In reality, "albumin" is a type of animal protein found in egg whites and in blood. "Albuminoids" are substances similar to "albumin".

assimilate/assimilation: It refers to the nutritional process by which food is transformed in the digestive system, it enters the blood flow and becomes part of the cells or serves as fuel for their functions.

biocatalyst: *See "catalyst"*.

biogur: A milk product of creamy consistency, made with *Streptococcus termophillus* and *Lactobacillus acidophilus*, that looks and has the same nutritional properties as yogurt, but is more readily assimilated due to the type of lactic acid it contains.

cardiovascular: From *kardia*, "heart", in Greek, and "vascular", which refers to blood vessels. It alludes to the heart and all the blood vessels within the circulatory system.

catalyst: Substance which does not integrate the final product of a chemical reaction, but which is needed –usually in small amounts– for the reaction to take place. Vitamins and oligoelements act as "catalysts". Organic catalysts are usually called "biocatalysts" (from *bios*, "life" in Greek.)

chemical substance: Any product in a pure state, be it natural or artificial (see chemical).

chemical compound: See "chemical".

chemical/chemistry: Refers to the composition of natural or artificial products. When dealing with chemical reactions of living organisms, the term "biochemistry" is sometimes used.

cottage cheese: A product of a creamy consistency and mild flavor, used by separating the proteins in milk serum. It is generally healthier and easier to digest than cured cheeses, due to its low fat content. Sometimes incorrectly used to refer to "fresh cheese" (see).

CSIC, Consejo Superior de Investigaciones Cientificas: Spain's national board for scientific research.

curd: Coagulated milk, not by "lactic fermentation", but by "enzymatic action" such as in the process for making cheese. Its consistency, nutritional value and use are similar to those of yogurt. In some places the term may refer to "fresh cheese" or "cottage cheese".

diet: Synonym with "regimen" or weight-loss plans. In this book it generally refers to the "form or method of eating".

dry fruits: Fruits which are usually eaten in their fresh state, but are dried for conserving. Its nutrients become concentrated from the loss of water. Common dry fruits include raisins, prunes, dry figs, peaches and nectarines. Not to be confused with dry oleaginous products.

dry oleaginous products: Refers to almonds, pecans, peanuts, pistachios, Brazil nuts, etc. Referred to generically as "nuts", sometimes called "fruits", although they are essentially seeds which grow inside a fruit.

enzyme: A substance which serves as a catalyst in the chemical reactions which take place within living organisms. Sometimes referred to as "fermenting" agents.

FAO: Food and Agriculture Organization of the United Nations.

fecula: Starch (see p. 39) obtained from roots, tubers or rhyzomes or plants such as potato, yams, cassava, or from some cereals such as corn. In many countries, cornstarch is the most popular fecula. Fecula is a refined product, and as such it is usually a pure carbohydrate, practically exempt of vitamins or minerals.

ferment: Agent producing fermentation. Older term for enzyme.

flakes: Pre-cooked and flattened whole cereals. Although some cereals may be ready to eat, some whole grain flakes need to be cooked further or soaked before eating.

"foie gras", vegetable: A kind of vegetable paté, made as a substitute for the popular French *foie gras*, which is made –as its name implies (from *foie*, "liver", and *gras*, "fat")– from the liver of fattened pigs or geese. The true "foie gras" is highly undesirable as a source of healthful nutrition.

food yeast: An excellent source of protein and vitamins, especially of the B complex. It is a highly useful nutritional complement. Different types are: "brewer's yeast" (see p. 146), and "lactic" yeast. They may be "stabilized" and processed to counter their bitterness, or as a basic component of several products.

fresh cheese: That which has only suffered lactic fermentation. It is characterized by a white color, soft texture and mild taste. Salt is usually added to retard spoilage. Its fat content is very low.

garden produce: Any food product which can be grown in a garden, including vegetables, legumes and tubers (potatoes, yams, etc.).

germ: Part of the grain or seed of cereals which contain all the vital elements for reproduction or "germination" of the plant (see sprouts). Because it contains germinal cells, it is a food with exceptional nutritional qualities. It is usually eliminated from the grain to avoid spoilage. It can be found in health food stores as a nutritional complement (see p. 146).

germs: In plural, it usually refers to microorganisms which can produce diseases. Sometimes referred to as "pathogens".

glucids: Synonym for "carbohydrate" (See p. 37).

gluten: Wheat protein, extracted by elimination of the starch. Used as a substitute for meat, sometimes mixed with soy protein (see "vegetarian meats").

greens: In the area of nutrition or dietetics it refers to those plant products that have edible green leaves, raw or cooked, such as: lettuce, escarole, cabbage, chard, spinach, etc. (see "garden produce").

hydrosoluble: That which can be dissolved in water. For example, vitamins B and C. As opposed to "liposoluble" (see further).

integral: Refers to a food (cereal, bread, sugar) which has not been refined, and as such keeps all its elements and original nutritional qualities. Integral products are many times called "whole" (see), and in some cases (whole wheat bread, sugar) are known as "black".

legumes: It generally refers to all types of fruit or seed found inside a pod and used when dry. For example, peas are usually considered a vegetable when fresh, and a legume when dry. Common legumes are: beans, lentils, garbanzos, lima beans, peas and soybeans.

lipid: Synonym of fat (see p. 45).

liposoluble: It may be dissolved in fat or oil; for instance, vitamins A, D, E and K. As opposed to hydrosoluble (see).

metabolism/metabolyze: The total of chemical processes by which the body assimilates, utilizes and eliminates the substances it ingests.

mineral salts: Minerals which have nutritional value are generally found in the form of chemical salts. Table salt is a "mineral salt" made up of sodium and chloride.

minerals: Inorganic products the body needs for proper functioning. They are considered nutrients (see). They are calcium, potassium, iron, magnesium, sodium, etc. Minerals which are needed in very small portions are called "oligoelements" (see).

molasses: Sweet product of similar consistency to honey made from sugar cane syrup after the crystallized sugar has been removed. It contains 60% saccarose and glucose, but it has more minerals (potassium, calcium and magnesium) and vitamins than brown sugar, and in many aspects is as good or better than honey.

molecule: In chemistry it refers to the smallest part of a substance which retains all of its qualities. Chemical formulas show the elements and the number of atoms each has, which make up the molecule. For instance, the chemical formula for water, H_2O, indicates that each of its molecules is made up of two atoms of hydrogen and one of oxygen.

muesli: German word referring to a breakfast cereal consumed in the nordic countries and central Europe. It is a mix of cereal flakes, dry fruits and nuts (see). It is a healthful and complete food that may be mixed with milk or yogurt, honey or molasses (see). It may be prepared at home or bought in processed form in stores.

nutrient: A substance needed to sustain human life. Main nutrients are carbohydrates, proteins and fats. Vitamins, minerals and even water are considered "nutrients."

oligoelements: A word referring to inorganic substances our bodies need in very small amounts (*oligos* is a Greek word meaning "little bit") for proper functioning, such as cobalt or nickel; which in larger amounts could even result toxic. All oligoelements are minerals.

parasitosis: Diseases provoked by "parasites", that is, organisms which live inside another and derive sustenance from it. Trichina is a parasite which lives inside the muscles of its host. Pinworms live inside the intestines, same as the flatworm.

pathologic: medical term (from *pathos*, "disease", and *logos*, "study of") which refers to "diseases", or "that which causes it", or to any morbid state.

protein/proteid: Synonyms used to refer to that which is related to proteins.

regimen: In nutrition it refers to the method of eating and as a synonym of "diet" (see). Sometimes used in the sense of imposing restrictions for healing purposes.

sanogur: Name given in some countries to a number of milk products similar to yogurt.

skim: Milk whose fat or cream has been extracted, partially (sometimes labeled 2%, 1% fat milk), or totally (nonfat or skim milk).

soy milk: A drink made from soy to which calcium and vitamins can be added, creating a product that may substitute for cow's milk with the advantage of not having any cholesterol or saturated fats (see p. 153).

sprouts: To obtain maximum nutritional benefits, cereal and legumes may be allowed to germinate in a wet environment. Alfalfa and soybean sprouts can be found in health food stores and some supermarkets.

synthesize: In chemistry and biochemistry it refers to uniting two or more elements or compounds, to form a new substance. "Chemical synthesis" is a process which can be either natural or artificial.

vegetable paté: A paste made with vegetable products which can be spread over other foods or bread (see "foie gras").

vegetable sausage: That which is made with "vegetarian meat" (see).

vegetarian burger: Made with vegetable protein.

vegetarian meat: A product usually made with soy protein, which in some cases may contain dry grains or nuts, flour, and gluten. "Vegetarian meat" products provide complete protein, and can be used as a healthy substitute for "animal meat", especially in a transition from an omnivorous to a vegetarian diet (see pages 166, 171). There are several manufacturers of vegetarian meat in Europe and the Americas.

WHO: World Health Organization. A worldwide medical and public health authority funded by the United Nations. Its public health journal *World Health* is published in several languages.

whole: 1. When used regarding foods, it is a synonym for "integral" (see). **2.** In the case of milk, "whole" milk contains all its fat, as opposed to nonfat or skim milk (see). **3.** It may refer to such food, diet or nutritional plan which provides all basic nutrients. Eggs and milk, although debatable, are considered "whole" foods. **4.** "Whole protein" is that which contains all "essential amino acids" and in the ideal proportion (see pages 60, 61).

yogurt: A milk product of creamy consistency, easy to digest and with an acidic flavor. It is made by fermentation with *Streptococcus termophillus* and *Lactobacillus bulgarius* (see "biogur", and "curd").

ILLUSTRATIONS

All **photographs, charts, graphs** and **drawings** not listed below have been created by **SAFELIZ EDITORIAL TEAM** (see page 4).

COREL: pages 14, 15, 16, 25, 40, 84, 104, 120, 121, 123, 124, 126, 127, 136, 156, 160.

DIGITAL VISION: pages 12, 114.

GRANOVITA: pages 144, 147, 149, 166.

HERNANDEZ, ANDRÉS: page 15.

INDEX: cover and page 28.

LIFE ART: pages 116, 117, 118, 121.

LOMA LINDA UNIVERSITY: page 111.

MINISTERY OF AGRICULTURE OF SPAIN: page 135.

NAENNY, EDOUARD: page 43.

PAMPLONA-ROGER, JORGE D.: pages 17, 18, 39, 42, 46, 47, 52, 59, 66, 68, 75, 83, 88, 92, 106, 107, 108, 133, 152.

PHOTODISC: pages 14, 17, 19, 26, 27, 29, 36, 44, 54, 64, 85, 87, 94, 96, 102, 119, 125, 128, 151, 157, 158, 170.

SANITARIUM HEALTH FOOD COMPANY, Nutrition Education Service: back cover and pages 14, 16, 41, 57, 60, 63, 93, 141, 172, 173.

STOCKBYTE: back cover and pages 9, 19, 22, 71.

TEJEL ALMORÍN, ANDRÉS: pages 32, 50, 61, 69, 70, 72, 73, 76, 79, 84, 89, 90, 131 ,148, 168, 169.

WERNER, LUDWIG: pages 30, 101, 154, 162, 163, 175.

UNITS OF MEASURE

USED IN THIS BOOK

calorie: Unit of energy. In general, when we talk about calories, we refer to «kilocalories». A calorie is the amount of heat (energy) needed to raise the temperature of a liter of water by one degree centigrade in normal atmospheric conditions. A kcal is equal to 4.18 kj (kilojoules); which means that to convert from kcal into kj, one only needs to multiply the amount by 4.18.

cc: Cubic centimeters are not used very often for the measurement of liquids. A «cubic centimeter» equals exactly a milliliter (ml).

cl: Centiliter, one-hundreth of a liter. 1 l = 100 cl.

dl: Deciliter, a liquid measure equal to one-tenth liter.

g: Symbol of "gram". A unit of weight in the metric system equalling a thousandth of a kilogram. 1 g = 0.001 kg.

kg: Symbol of "kilogram" or "kilo". One kilogram equals one thousand grams.

kj: Symbol of "kilojoule."

joule: Measure of energy used in the English system. As it happens with the "calorie", kilojoule is more commonly used. Chemists and physicists often prefer "joules" to "calories" when measuring energy. A kj equals 0.24 kcal; which means that, in order to convert kj into kcal, one needs to multiply the amount by 0.24.

I.U.: International Units, a unit of measurement that was employed when the weight of some vitamins could not be measured exactly. It is a measure of the "biological effects" of a substance upon living organisms. Today, micrograms is a more common unit of measurement (µg). In the case of vitamin A: 1 µg = 3.33 I.U.

l: Symbol of "liter", unit of liquid measure in the metric system. 1 l = 1 dm^3 = 1,000 cc = 1,000 ml.

mcg: Sometimes used as the symbol for "microgram". The international symbol µg is preferred (see).

mg: Symbol of milligram, equal to one-thousandth of a gram. 1 g = 1,000 mg.

ml: Symbol of milliliter, a thousandth of a liter: 1 l = 1,000 ml (1 ml = 1 cc).

µg: Symbol of microgram, a thousandth of a milligram: 1 mg = 1,000 µg.

RE: Retinol Equivalent, see I.U.

The information provided in this work on the composition of foods is based on data published by the United States Department of Agriculture, AH-8 issue 11 (http://www.nal.usda.gov/fnic/foodcomp).

The recommended daily amounts (RDA) are those established by the US National Research Council in 1989, 10th edition. National Academy of Sciences, Washington DC.

INDEX

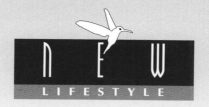

NEW LIFESTYLE

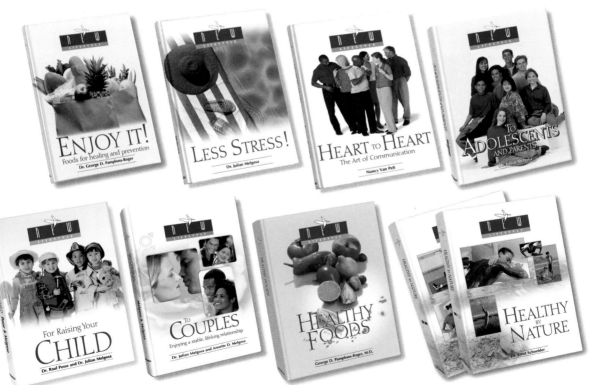